JOURNEY TO HEALING

THE ART AND SCIENCE OF APPLIED KINESIOLOGY

EUGENE CHARLES, D.C.

Renaissance Publishers, 115 Ardmore Avenue, Melville, NY 11747

All names of patients have been changed to protect their privacy.

As with any serious medical conditions, readers are advised to consult with a physician regarding their health and treatment.

Printed in the United States of America
Library of Congress Control Number: 2019931252

ISBN 978-0-9644217-6-9

To Donna

TABLE OF CONTENTS

APPENDICES

ACKNOWLEDGMENTS

Much of the historical information came from personal conversations with Dr. George Goodheart when we would engage in our long talks every year celebrating our mutual birthday. His brilliance created a ripple that continues to grow and was the spark that ignited this book.

I am indebted to Mrs. Joanne Goodheart, Dr. Robert Blaich, Dr. Walter Schmitt, Dr. Sheldon Deal, Dr. Martin Rosen, Dr. Stephen Press, and Dr. Donald McDowell for helping me to "fill in the historical blanks."

I am grateful to my editor, Paul Dinas, who helped turn a doctor into a writer and then a writer into an author.

I acknowledge my Applied Kinesiology colleagues, who work day-in and day-out to relieve so much pain and suffering. You are an indispensable guide in your patient's journey to healing.

To you—the reader. Never stop believing that you can be better. Your health is the motivating reason why doctors learn the art and science of Applied Kinesiology.

Most of all, I thank my wife, Donna, with all my heart. Your love, support, and dedication provided me with the faith to make *Journey to Healing* a reality.

FOREWORD

Dr. Eugene Charles has been one of the premier instructors in the field of Applied Kinesiology (AK) for over three decades. Chiropractors, osteopaths and physicians like myself have all appreciated his fund of knowledge and mastery of AK as developed by the late great George Goodheart. Not only is he a phenomenal instructor but also a consummate clinician, who in this work has provided a full-on display of the applications of AK. This is a work that should turn heads and stimulate a genuine interest among primary care clinicians across all disciplines. The only people who will be more excited are those suffering from ailments that have not been helped or fully helped by allopathic and traditional manipulative therapies. AK offers a real alternative.

Applied Kinesiology is one of the greatest medical diagnostic and therapeutic systems to become available to practitioners in recent times. While many of you reading this may not be aware of this therapeutic system, I guarantee that you will want to know more as you read Dr. Charles' clear exposition of the roots of this system of healing, its development, and applications. As you will learn, the real instructor in Applied Kinesiology is the body itself. No need for a poor animal in a laboratory or a clinical drug trial. At least two generations of chiropractors and osteopaths have added to the growing knowledge of functional anatomy and body energetics. In a medical landscape dominated by high tech medical applications, AK gets back to basics, addressing everyday musculoskeletal problems and beyond, without using aggressive drugs and often avoiding the need for surgical intervention.

Clinicians will appreciate the wide range of therapeutic applications of Applied Kinesiology. Moreover, all of this work is rooted in clinical observation and tried and true methodologies that have proven efficacy. Mainstream medical science has not been forsaken in AK. Rather, the gaping holes in functional assessments of problems are overcome by an AK analysis, and, in many cases, an enhanced understanding of the problem leads to new and more efficacious treatment options. If five clinicians trained in AK were to see the same patient, they could all use the same techniques and achieve the same result. On the other hand, five people with the same named illness may require five different ways to approach their problem.

The training in this discipline is very hands on. It's about working with live bodies. As a traditionally trained physician, I loved this about my training in AK. I got to directly experience the benefits of this work as fellow practitioners workshopped on each other and now with the advent of DVD and online classes, of immediately implementing the procedures on my patients. Applied Kinesiology requires an intimate knowledge of the functional anatomy of the body and brings into play other disciplines beyond Western medicine. The results that can be achieved as a clinician using this discipline will make your day an extremely gratifying one and endear you to your patients. The journey of practitioners, from applying set protocols for problems faced in their daily medical practice, to really having the tools to uncover what is at the root of the body's dysfunction, will be greatly served by mastering this discipline.

For the general public and allied health professionals reading this book, you will appreciate the actual real-life stories of patients, with common problems that you have probably had contact with and/or can personally relate to, being helped by an AK intervention. While there may be presentations of patients with the same clinical diagnosis, Dr. Charles will clearly reveal how an AK assessment goes beyond the standard convention of labeling a dysfunction and treating the label and not the person. No one technique fixes all in AK. Everyone is an individual on their own particular path; developing problems not in a vacuum, but in the context of their lives. All health is relational, and AK expands the understanding of what must be appreciated to bring a client to cure.

I believe that the public will appreciate this discipline in the context of figuring out what kind of health care they want to receive for themselves and where AK might fit in. The Applied Kinesiologist is indeed "the body whisperer," and this discipline will add to anyone's understanding of what is actually going on with his or her body. As you scan the chapter headings, you will see the wide variety of problems that are successfully addressed with non-invasive AK procedures. This work reflects Dr. Charles' clinical prowess and years of refinement of his skills. Applied kinesiology is not a static discipline, and Dr. Charles has added to the body of clinical knowledge that constitutes Applied Kinesiology. I want to pull out a passage that appears early in *Journey to Healing*:

"Applied Kinesiology's unique system of Functional Muscle Testing (FMT) is an interactive assessment tool that measures physiological health at that precise moment of the test. The muscle test, as performed in AK, is a window into the central integrative state of the person's nervous system and its neural pathways. It is a diagnostic tool that evaluates the physiological status of the motor neurons, as well as their proper function and relation to the muscles and other systems of the body. Muscles, bones, nerves, fascia, and organs are interconnected and codependent. When one specific muscle is not functioning properly, it can affect one's entire system."

This is the core concept in Applied Kinesiology. The closest you can come to approximating such an understanding of the body would be through the pulse-taking of Chinese medicine, and here you would have needed years of mentorship. What Applied Kinesiology offers is an interactive system that is in the moment, with instantaneous change possible as techniques are applied. Both the client and the practitioner can determine at the moment if progress has been made! This can be done without introducing a substance into the body and even before the results of lab and radiologic tests are available. This is a game changer for both practitioner and patient.

Seeing the display of applied kinesiological assessment and therapeutic processes in this work, I can only hope that Dr. Charles will continue to write and teach as he receives the praise and accolades he deserves from fellow practitioners and the public for sharing such a clear exposition of a true healing discipline.

Kamau Kokayi, M.D.

INTRODUCTION

True health is not simply the absence of disease. It is a state of being in which the miraculous physical and mental forces that make us human work together in proper balance. True health allows us to be ourselves and live every day at our own personal best. Achieving true health is a journey—unique to every individual.

However, many of us do not feel the need to begin this journey until we experience symptoms, such as pain or dysfunction, that interfere with our quality of life. The disruption of our health becomes something that needs to be "fixed." So we visit our doctors in the hope of finding relief. Traditional mainstream medicine, while immensely helpful in combatting disease and medical conditions, neglects the deeper concept of true health by treating the condition and its symptoms, not the total individual. Under our present system, doctors simply do not have the time to evaluate the overall health of their patients. Therefore, they are forced to focus on the specific symptom or condition, instead of trying to find the underlying source of the problem and treating it with an appropriate therapy to heal the entire body.

The fundamental weakness in this approach is that it doesn't help the patient achieve true health. It applies general therapeutic procedures proven to address the condition, not the person. Often, what might be an effective treatment for one person might not prove as effective for another with the same condition because of their unique physiology and circumstances. Many patients might get temporary relief, but the underlying imbalance in their system tends to resurface in the future. As a result, too many people end the journey to healing before it has truly begun and never achieve optimal and lasting health.

Applied Kinesiology (AK) follows a different model. It is the science of healing the total person and supporting his or her true health through the study of movement and integral muscle function. Patients often visit an AK specialist after they have run the gamut of traditional medical professionals with little or no success. AK specialists take the time to do an extensive interview with each patient to assess his or her concerns regarding their health. They review the results of any standard tests the patient has undergone. Then, by observing how a person moves and subsequently testing various muscles by hand that are linked to a particular condition or symptom, the Applied Kinesiologist can create a unique treatment plan to alleviate the underlying dysfunction and restore the patient to health.

Applied Kinesiology utilizes a spectrum of noninvasive diagnostic and treatment protocols to restore optimal function to your body. These include various muscle manipulation techniques, chiropractic therapies, acupuncture, nutrition, cranial therapy, specific exercises, and mind/body procedures. Applied Kinesiology works on the subtle facets of your body that may not show up on traditional tests such as X-ray, MRI, CAT scans, or even blood work. Although these tests are useful in creating a full patient profile, they are somewhat static in nature—like snapshots of a person's physiology. By their very nature of being more structurally rather than *functionally* oriented, these tests do not necessarily reveal the dysfunction in the inner dynamics of your body that may be the actual source of the problem. Many patients who have undergone these tests received "normal" results but still feel horrible.

In contrast, AK testing is more like a motion picture, capturing the synergistic functions of the body as a whole. It looks beyond the limitations of strictly empirical evidence to discover the problem and restores balance and optimal function in your body.

My own personal connection to AK began nearly four decades ago. At that time, I had been suffering from severe shoulder pain since my teenage years due to a sports-related injury. The pain was so severe that I could not exercise or pursue sports. I'd been to many medical professionals and chiropractic doctors over the years but could not find relief.

Having been helped by doctors of chiropractic for previous injuries, I decided to become a chiropractor. Along with helping others, I was hoping that I would finally find a solution to my problem—so I matriculated at The Los Angeles College of Chiropractic. In my second term, I was perplexed and frustrated that, despite my training, I could not find the source of my condition. Not even my experienced teachers could help relieve my pain. A classmate told me about a cutting-edge discipline known as Applied Kinesiology. Though it was not taught at chiropractic schools at the time, it had the reputation of being miraculous for its ability to tap the body's innate healing power. I saw some impressive demonstrations of AK by upper classmates and became intrigued. As it happened, the founder of AK, Dr. George Goodheart, was giving a weekend seminar nearby. I decided that I would go to the source to learn more about it. Little did I know that it would be a life-changing experience for me.

At the seminar, Dr. Goodheart spoke about many conditions that could be helped with AK methodologies. I listened intently as he said, "Athletes are finely tuned and need to be finely treated." Then he specifically talked about how this new approach could dramatically help with athletic injuries. I was thoroughly impressed by the depth of his knowledge, as well as by his humility about what he had discovered.

After the presentation, I went up to him and shared the story about my ongoing shoulder condition. He listened intensely and then asked three specific questions: how it began, where the pain was localized, and what treatments I had undergone. After hearing my "case history," Dr. Goodheart observed my posture and then had me walk, noting that my arm remained constantly pinned to my side. He performed a muscle test on one of my shoulder muscles (deltoid), and it was painful and weak. He proceeded to stabilize a joint in my shoulder, where the collar bone and shoulder blade meet, by holding the joint together with his one hand and again tested the muscle with his other hand. The muscle now tested stronger and was much less painful.

Literally, within minutes, he diagnosed the mysterious source of my problem: a slightly separated acromioclavicular joint detectable only through functional muscle testing (FMT) and a procedure known as Extremity Challenging—both specific to AK.

Dr. Goodheart suggested that I see a local doctor who was at the seminar and well-trained in AK. Perhaps sensing my disappointment, Goodheart (as he would later tell me) broke protocol. Right on the conference floor, he gave me a light chiropractic adjustment to realign the shoulder joint. I felt relief for the first time in years. He then offered advice as to what my classmates, who were with me at the seminar, could do to accelerate the healing process for the strained joint; namely muscle manipulation techniques, precise chiropractic adjustments, how to tape the shoulder properly, some specific exercises to follow, and changes in my diet and nutrition. I took detailed notes and left with hope for relief.

Within three months of Dr. Goodheart's initial evaluation and treatment, along with the additional treatments and advice he recommended, I was completely cured of my shoulder pain. I had begun my journey to true health and continue on its path to this day. Ever since this personal experience of being healed by AK, I have been inspired by the potential of Applied Kinesiology to improve people's lives and have made it my life's work.

Applied Kinesiology is a unique healing system that any doctor or health care professional can incorporate into his or her practice. However, very few doctors and even fewer patients are aware of this amazingly effective approach to helping people with a wide variety of health conditions. I have treated well over 6,000 patients and have taught thousands of doctors from many specialties in the art and science of AK. Yet AK remains virtually unknown to the vast majority of people, many of whom may be suffering needlessly. My motivation for writing this book is to rectify that lack of familiarity, as well as to clarify any misinformation that has circulated about it.

Progressive MDs are well aware that something is missing in Western medicine, and, as the US life expectancy continues to drop in significant segments of the population, doctors are now opening up to embrace AK, which at first appears to be a seemingly inexplicable healing system. Reminiscent of the stories of

Dr. Joseph Lister (of Listerine® fame) and Florence Nightingale, both of whom were at first scoffed at by colleagues for suggesting that doctors and nurses wash their hands before surgery, there is a burgeoning of intuitive doctors enthusiastic to learn something new and yet paradoxically old. This is encouraging because, along with the declining lifespan of the general population,[1] physician dissatisfaction, burnout, and suicide rate are becoming alarmingly high.[2] Perhaps engaging in the exciting field of AK may benefit physicians nearly as much as patients.

It seems that, to make a profound change in the healthcare of people worldwide, more medical doctors need to start implementing this holistic method of diagnosis and treatment into their practice. Why? Simple mathematics. For example, in the USA, there are essentially 1,000,000 medical doctors and approximately 50,000 doctors of chiropractic in a country with a population of nearly 330,000,000. The only way AK can make a meaningful change in the health of America is for medical doctors to jump on board and incorporate this powerful healing tool into their private practices. Doctors who are interested in adding AK to their practice can learn from live classes through the International College of Applied Kinesiology (ICAK)[3,4] and online classes[5,6]

In these pages, I have included case histories of patients' experiences with AK. Many of these people had nearly given up hope to ever live *normal* lives again until treatments with AK restored their true health and put them back on their personal journey to healing. I hope that their stories will inspire you about the power of AK to help you to reach your full health potential and set you on your own lifelong journey to healing.

PART I

APPLIED KINESIOLOGY AND ITS COMMITMENT TO HEALTH

1

A BRIEF HISTORY OF APPLIED KINESIOLOGY

As with many groundbreaking medical discoveries, AK started with a new perspective on an age-old challenge to doctors everywhere: to relieve pain and achieve optimal health in their patients.

Dr. George Goodheart, Sr., was a successful chiropractic doctor in Detroit, Michigan in the 1920s. Chiropractic was a relatively new science at the time, having been founded in 1895 by Daniel David Palmer. It grew in popularity but remained controversial. The traditional medical doctors denounced it as lacking in scientific validity, despite the massive amount of practical research it had garnered. Yet men like Goodheart, who were committed to healing through the innate mechanisms of the human body, followed its precepts and helped hundreds of people.

Dr. Goodheart incorporated a well-rounded approach to patient care. He was constantly looking for better ways to serve his patients. He would travel around the Midwest to meet with other innovative doctors in the chiropractic profession, often bringing his son, George Jr. with him. One such individual, who recalled young George visiting his lab in knee pants with his father, was the brilliant doctor, "Major" Bertrand DeJarnette. Dr. DeJarnette discovered a technique called Sacro-Occipital Technique (SOT) that became one of the most respected techniques in chiropractic.

Influenced by his respect for his father's passion for healing people, George Goodheart Jr. followed in his father's footsteps and studied to become a chiropractic doctor. After attending the University of Detroit, he went on to graduate from The National College of Chiropractic in 1939 and planned to join his father's successful practice. The Second World War interrupted his plan, however. After serving with distinction in The United States Air Corps, he returned home to begin his work with his father in 1946.

Brimming with enthusiasm to heal the sick, the young doctor would often ask his father how to handle particularly difficult cases. The senior Dr. Goodheart would urge him to rely on his intuition to solve the problem. He advised him always "to see with eyes that truly see; hear with ears that truly hear; feel with hands that truly feel."

After his father's death, Dr. Goodheart continued to practice as he had done for nearly two decades. However, in 1964, he made a groundbreaking discovery. A 24-year-old man came to his office with excruciating shoulder pain. He complained that he'd been to many doctors, but no one could help him. His condition was compounded by an inability to push forward with the arm affected by the shoulder pain.

Dr. Goodheart did a thorough examination of the patient to discover that one of his shoulder blades protruded prominently, causing it to be unstable. This condition is known as a "winging scapula." Goodheart had some X-rays taken. The films showed that there was no deformity in the bones themselves or misalignment. Goodheart was unable to alleviate this man's shoulder pain and weakness using the usual therapeutic options available to him.

Unwilling to accept his inability to help this man, Dr. Goodheart redoubled his efforts to find a solution. As a student of all past and present developments in his profession, just as his father had been, he turned to the landmark text *Muscles: Testing and Function*, written by two pioneering physical therapists, the husband and wife team of Henry and Florence Kendall in 1949. Expanding on the work of Dr. Robert W. Lovett, a professor of orthopedic surgery at Harvard University who is credited with first utilizing muscle testing techniques to help polio victims, the Kendalls shared their insights into the impact of weak muscles on the general well-being of the body's mechanical systems and introduced relatively new techniques of musculoskeletal examination and treatment.

Goodheart surmised that a weakness in the *serratus anterior* muscle on the chest wall that normally pulls the shoulder blade forward could be the source of his patient's problem. The Kendalls reported that it could be tested for strength by having the patient stand and face a wall. Then the patient would lift both arms and put his or her hands on the wall. Once in position, the patient would press forward on the wall. If the shoulder blade stuck out, it meant that the muscle was weak. Goodheart performed the muscle test on his patient and found this to be the case. But what was causing the weakness and how could he alleviate it?

Goodheart examined the muscle and found what felt to be small nodules in the muscle itself. Nodules, commonly known as "trigger points," had been discussed in articles in medical journals, predominantly by Janet Travell, M.D.—White House Physician to Presidents John F. Kennedy and Lyndon B. Johnson. As early as 1946, Travell had discovered that these nodules, also known as myofascial adhesions, caused pain and dysfunction in the muscle and would often refer pain to other areas. At the time, the nodules were treated principally with anesthetic injections to numb the pain and dissipate the myofascial adhesions. What Goodheart actually found appeared to be a "knot" within the muscle itself, separate from the nodules that Travell discovered that were located in the *covering* of the muscle (fascia).

This was new therapeutic territory for Goodheart. The knots in his patient's muscle appeared to be the source of his muscular weakness. He followed his intuition and manipulated the muscle, effectively rubbing the knots out of the muscle. After this procedure, the man moved his shoulder and arm and said that his pain was almost gone. Goodheart then had the man perform the Kendall's medical muscle test again. To Goodheart's amazement, the shoulder blade now barely stuck out, and the patient's arm strength came back. The dysfunction had largely disappeared—along with the pain and the nodule. His patient was cured in an almost miraculous way. The young man thanked him profusely and left.

Goodheart was dumbfounded. This flew in the face of conventional wisdom. In his experience, muscles took weeks, often months, of careful *spinal manipulation* and *exercise* to regain strength and function properly. How could a muscle respond so quickly to a few minutes of simple *muscle manipulation*?

Upon further analysis, Goodheart concluded that slight tears in the muscle, known as microavulsions, could theoretically cause a buildup of muscle waste products such as lymphatics and lactic acid to create nodules in the muscle. These nodules differed from the well-documented Travell trigger points because these points did not refer (transmit) pain to other regions of the body, and these *new* nodules were located deeper within the muscle itself and not the overlying fascial covering.

Theoretically, these nodules that Goodheart discovered either caused or were the result of a communication error between the nerves and the muscle at the neuromuscular junction—creating its dysfunction and effectively "shutting off" the related muscle. The Golgi tendon organ (GTO) is the sensory receptor that senses how much tension is in the tendon when a muscle is contracting. If there is too much muscle tension, the GTO will inhibit the muscle from creating any force—demonstrating as *weakness* on muscle testing—to protect the muscle from further injuring itself. This leads to the *shutting off* of the muscle. Massaging out the nodules reset the Golgi tendon organ nerve endings, restoring normal function and allowing the muscle waste to freely flow out of the muscles and into the lymphatic drainage system. This relieved the blockage and restored normal neural impulses, thus allowing the muscle to function properly almost immediately.

Dr. Goodheart sensed that he had inadvertently discovered an entirely new approach to muscle testing. Up to this point, the results of muscle strength testing were thought to be static—like seeing a fracture on an X-ray. Goodheart's breakthrough was that muscle "weakness" was not necessarily a *pathological* problem, but a *physiological* one. For example, a weakness found when muscle testing could be due to a severe muscle tear which represents a pathological problem and usually requires surgery. Goodheart's discovery uncovered that slight tears, such as in the above initial discovery, represent a *physiological weakness* and can be corrected non-surgically with an immediate and measurable improvement in muscle function.

Therefore, manual muscle testing could be a diagnostic tool as a dynamic measure of relative function rather than disability. Goodheart magnified the depth of the meaning of the muscle test similar to what a microscope did to the magnifying glass; it revealed more of what was happening deep in the physiology of the person. This original technique of manually manipulating the Golgi tendon organs located at both ends of the muscle to restore normal function to a muscle became known as Origin/Insertion Technique. This procedure has since become the standard AK treatment in cases of muscular dysfunction due to traumatic injuries.

This case brought to Goodheart's attention the fact that painful conditions are often caused not only by misalignment of the spine or other bone structures but also by weakness or physiological inhibition in the muscles that hold them in place. Since muscles move bones, they need to be functioning properly to keep the bone and joint structure in proper alignment. This represented an advanced and, arguably, an inverted approach to chiropractic therapy; i.e., to maintain optimum joint alignment, doctors would need to *manipulate muscles* first.

Goodheart began introducing this new approach to muscle testing into his practice and experienced even greater success than he had before his discovery. However, he found that many patients actually experienced muscle weakness (physiological inhibition) without nodules. Goodheart learned that the nodules were only present in cases of trauma, signaling the need for the Origin/Insertion Technique. He then found other factors that could cause muscle inhibition, such as Travell's trigger points that only weaken a muscle after it is stretched. This meant that the key lay in the muscle test, not the palpable nodules. Intrigued by other possible causes of *physiological* muscle weakness, Dr. Goodheart began to scour all the available literature on innovative techniques by chiropractors, osteopaths, and medical doctors and attempted a wide variety of procedures to expand his ability to heal his patients.

Dr. Goodheart developed a new, multi-disciplinary, and integrative system that drew upon such diverse healthcare systems as chiropractic, osteopathic, acupuncture, massage, nutrition, and psychology as well as traditional medicine. Manual muscle testing became the gateway diagnostic tool to find the most appropriate treatment to restore the total health of his patients, not just alleviate their specific complaints.

Excited by his discoveries, he began sharing his findings with local chiropractors, who would meet regularly with Goodheart in his downtown Detroit office and later in Gaylord, Michigan. After applying Goodheart's techniques, many of the visiting chiropractors reported similarly dramatic results.

He decided to call this system "Applied Kinesiology." Kinesiology is from the Greek *kinesis*, which means motion or movement. Kinesiology essentially means "the study of muscular movement especially the mechanics of human motion." At the time, while the science of kinesiology was beginning to be well established, it was primarily an academic discipline. Kinesiologists had been around since at least 1926 when a group of physical education specialists founded the Academy of Kinesiology and Physical Education. They conducted research and held forums to share their findings with a wide variety of medical professionals at the time, but kinesiology was not perceived as a diagnostic technique for general health.

Hence, Goodheart's addition of the word "Applied" underscored its practical use in the treatment of patients. Goodheart believed that he had discovered a practical way to diagnose, measure and treat bodily dysfunction via the muscular system. While AK began as a subspecialty within the chiropractic profession, it developed into an innovative healing discipline that uses the chiropractic adjustment as one of its many powerful tools.

Goodheart began publishing his findings in yearly AK manuals as well as chiropractic journals. He also continued to spread the word about this new discipline by lecturing to medical professionals around the country. Goodheart, eager to share this knowledge, accepted speaking engagements nationwide at state and national conventions sponsored by chiropractic organizations. His presentations were received with enthusiasm.

However, many doctors often were not able to reproduce the results that Dr. Goodheart presented at the seminars. Goodheart decided to change the venue from a lecture, where he would simply discuss his findings, to hands-on workshops where doctors would break up into groups and work on each other. The new format was a success. Doctors reported an improved comprehension of the techniques and a greater number of positive outcomes with their patients.

As the success of the workshop method increased, more workshops by chiropractors teaching other chiropractors expanded. Eventually, Goodheart would appoint twelve study group leaders in various areas throughout the United States. This way, doctors interested in AK could learn the material that Goodheart had originally presented in a paced, hands-on style workshop without his having to be present. These workshop leaders would be affectionately labeled the original "Dirty Dozen" in the AK community.

Eventually, Goodheart realized the difficulty of personally supervising the workshop leaders and sharing the growing new research with them and decided to convert the group leaders into a formal organization. One of the workshop leaders, Dr. John Thie of Pasadena, California, encouraged this development and volunteered to put the first organizational meeting together.

In 1973, Goodheart and the original twelve workshop leaders, along with other doctors motivated to learn AK in a more structured setting, came together as an academic organization that would become The International College of Applied Kinesiology (ICAK). The ICAK was founded officially in 1975, and by 1976 the bylaws and its original officers were codified. A cohesive curriculum and a training system were established for doctors seeking to be certified AK practitioners—making AK part of their practices throughout the nation.

Workshop leaders gave way to teaching Diplomates who were responsible for training and referring new applicants for certification by the ICAK. In addition to teaching, the Diplomates were required to do research and publish papers in scientific journals.

Interested doctors and medical professionals paid annual dues and received regular updates in *The Proceedings of The ICAK,* a collection of case studies, research papers and new procedures for them to investigate and possibly utilize. Yearly meetings would showcase doctors sharing new techniques, theories and research. Often research in other disciplines published in scientific journals would be seamlessly integrated into new AK protocols. Applied Kinesiology was and remains a fluid system that seeks to improve and add healing techniques from a vast array of medical, scientific and holistic sources.

The yearlong (one hundred-hour) basic course was established as a postgraduate program for doctors to learn on weekends while they maintained their practices during the week. To support this initiative, Dr. David Walther of Pueblo, Colorado published the first of his seminal texts on AK in 1976 with the release of *Applied Kinesiology – The Advanced Approach in Chiropractic*. Dr. Walther also developed the original syllabus for the basic course, and other doctors would later contribute additional syllabuses and flowcharts to guide doctors through the ever-growing number of treatment options available.

The original AK course contained hundreds of techniques to teach doctors how to effectively help people with spinal problems, muscle pains, carpal tunnel syndrome, headaches, athletic injuries, digestive issues and, of course, shoulder problems—to name just a few. Once the medical professional completed the course successfully, he or she would receive official certification as a trained AK practitioner.

After doctors had studied for a minimum of three years and completed at least 300 hours of AK training, including the basic 100-hour course, they could be eligible for certification as a Diplomate of the International Board of Applied Kinesiology (DIBAK). The Diplomate program was instituted to develop criteria for advanced certification in the established and reproducible AK procedures which allowed the successful applicants to teach other medical professionals. Applicants had to be licensed doctors (DC, MD, DO) in practice for a minimum of three years and the authors of at least two original thesis papers. Once they passed the rigorous Diplomate Exam, they were certified by the ICAK as Diplomates—approved to teach other doctors the art and science of AK.

After the founding of the ICAK, Goodheart's success with AK continued to spread. His work was controversial, being praised as a breakthrough by many and criticized as unscientific by more traditionally entrenched physicians. Goodheart received numerous awards and distinctions throughout his lifetime. However, perhaps his proudest achievement was his appointment to the US Olympic Sports Medicine Committee as the first chiropractic physician to serve on the US Olympic Medical Team. Historically, chiropractors had been banned from being on the committee, even though most of the athletes had been treated by these practitioners privately for years and wanted them as part of the medical team.

Irving Dardik, M.D., a vascular surgeon, was the chairman of the United States Olympic Medical Committee for the 1980 Winter Games in Lake Placid, New York. Over the years, he had gone on record against the inclusion of chiropractic as part of the official Olympic medical service. This all changed when he would witness firsthand the power of AK and chiropractic.

Dr. Dardik, a world-class runner himself, developed a problem with his leg sometime in 1978. After a few miles of running, his hamstring would cramp up whenever he tried to pick up the pace and sprint. He visited some of the best sports doctors in the country, yet no one could figure out what the problem was. One of his colleagues suggested he contact Dr. Goodheart, a well-known doctor of chiropractic and the founder of AK.

Dardik was aware of this relatively new alternative discipline but remained skeptical about it. However, since he had run out of options regarding his mysterious leg cramping, plus the fact that America's best athletes were clamoring for an official team chiropractic physician, Dardik contacted Goodheart. Dr. Dardik wanted to learn more about this new discipline and its suitability for the Olympic team as well as to shed some light on his own condition.

Dr. and Mrs. Goodheart flew to New Jersey and met Dr. Dardik at his office. After a preliminary discussion, Dr. Dardik impressed upon Dr. Goodheart his mixed feelings about chiropractic in general and AK in particular. Not a stranger to this kind of attitude from the traditional medical community, Dr. Goodheart did his best to explain the science behind these two disciplines. Dr. Dardik was not convinced but was willing to learn more.

The meeting progressed from an interview to a consultation, when Dardik shared with Goodheart the additional reason he had contacted him—his leg pain. Goodheart listened intently and then explained how he would begin the examination, namely using the functional muscle testing procedures that he developed. Dardik, enthusiastic about this possibility, asked Goodheart if he could demonstrate and implement treatment immediately. Goodheart said it was irregular to administer a treatment without a more thorough examination, but he obliged.

In the office, Dr. Goodheart had Dr. Dardik lie on a large desk. Goodheart tested the hamstring muscle, and it tested strong. He then tested the calf muscle, and it too was strong. He proceeded to have Dr. Dardik flex the muscles of the foot and the opposite arm as if he was running and then immediately tested the calf. It became dramatically weak (physiologically inhibited). In other words, the hamstring and calf muscles were strong when tested in isolation. However, a calf weakness showed up only after contraction of the muscles on the foot and the opposite arm, which would naturally contract at the same time as the calf when walking or running. Often, running and sprinting puts so much strain on all these muscles that cramping can occur if there is dysfunction anywhere in the system.

Goodheart diagnosed the symptoms as caused by a *gait-mediated reactive muscle* condition and explained the problem to Dr. Dardik, who predictably had never heard of this condition. A gait-mediated reactive muscle condition occurs when the contraction of certain muscles during walking or running causes *excessive reciprocal inhibition* in a different muscle, resulting in the weakness of that muscle. In Dardik's case, the muscles and joint mechanoreceptors in the foot were inducing the calf to become weak (physiologically inhibited), subsequently causing the hamstring to eventually cramp up because it now had to work twice as hard without the help of the calf muscle.

The thorough explanation seemed to make sense to Dr. Dardik, and he asked what the treatment would entail. Dr. Goodheart explained that the treatment would involve the strict manipulation of the mechanoreceptors (sensory receptors that respond to mechanical pressure) located on the foot. Goodheart also explained that he would need to administer precise chiropractic adjustments to the metatarsal bones where the toes connect to the foot as well as to the calcaneal (heel) bone where the calf connects—all of which he found to be misaligned. Dardik agreed and, immediately following the treatment, he was now able to perform the calf muscle test after contracting his foot and opposite arm muscles easily. Goodheart instructed him to try running the next day to test out the effectiveness of the treatment.

Dr. Dardik thanked him for his work and told him he would be sure to let him know if his condition improved. He called a few days later to report that he had run farther than he had in some time with no pain or cramping.

Once he experienced for himself what a chiropractor using AK could achieve, he began to change his position regarding the inclusion of chiropractic for the Olympics. After discussing it with the other members of the committee, Dr. Goodheart was invited to Colorado Springs to describe in detail and demonstrate AK techniques to the other members of the United States Olympic Committee (USOC) Sports Medicine Council. Together with Dr. Dardik's testimony about how Dr. Goodheart had cured him of his perplexing condition, the USOC voted unanimously to offer the position to Dr. Goodheart to be The United States' first official team chiropractic physician. He accepted the offer, and the rest is history. Chiropractors have had an official place in the Olympic Games and greater prominence on professional sports teams ever since.

Over the years, some of the principal tributes and honors accumulated by Dr. Goodheart include Distinguished Service Awards from Palmer College of Chiropractic (1974, 1975), Elected Member of The American College of Sports Medicine (1984), Leonardo Da Vinci Award from The Institute for Achievement of Human Potential (1987), and Honoree from *Time* as one of the top 100 "Alternative Medicine Innovators" (2001).

Dr. George Goodheart died on March 5, 2008, at the age of 89. He is remembered as a tireless healing professional dedicated to the optimum health of his patients. He inspired thousands of men and women in the healing professions to employ AK. Since Goodheart's initial discovery in 1964, the International College of Applied Kinesiology (ICAK) has grown to become a nonprofit, worldwide, multidisciplinary organization with chapters throughout the world. It remains dedicated to research advancing manual muscle testing as a system of diagnosis for evaluating areas of dysfunction within the body. It is the principal organization for the training and certification for AK professionals, bringing together doctors of all disciplines with a common interest in using this powerful tool in the treatment of their patients.

Current estimates suggest that 1,000,000 practitioners worldwide are using some form of AK manual muscle testing,[7] and as more and more patients and medical professionals become aware of its benefits, this number will continue to climb. However, despite the world renown of its founder and his legacy, its continuing scientific research and meteoric growth as a powerful member of the functional medicine pantheon, AK, like many other nontraditional innovations in the field of medicine, remains plagued by controversy. As its benefits become more mainstream, it is only a matter of time before Applied Kinesiology takes its place as one of the most effective healthcare disciplines in the world today.

2

HOW APPLIED KINESIOLOGY WORKS

The premise of AK is simple: to allow the amazing curative powers of the human body to restore balance and achieve optimum health. The human body is a finely tuned system of complex checks and balances. When a condition arises that throws our body off, it can result in pain or illness. The goal of AK is to find the imbalance and help the body reset itself. Its principal diagnostic tool is a unique approach to diagnosing this imbalance by observing how a person moves in relation to the symptoms he or she might display. It might sound counterintuitive, but careful attention to a person's posture and movement is a vital diagnostic tool and represents an indication of muscle function that can reveal the source of the condition he or she has and how best to treat it.

Applied Kinesiology's unique system of Functional Muscle Testing (FMT) is an interactive assessment tool that measures physiological health at that precise moment of the test. The muscle test, as performed in AK, is a window into the central integrative state of the person's nervous system and its neural pathways. It is a diagnostic tool that evaluates the physiological status of the motor neurons, as well as their proper function and relation to the muscles and other systems of the body. Muscles, bones, nerves, fascia, and organs are interconnected and codependent. When one specific muscle is not functioning properly, it can affect one's entire system.

FMT can detect a neuromuscular dysfunction that may be due to *deafferentation,* or the loss of the normal messaging between receptors located in specific areas of the body and the nervous system. These receptors reside in muscles, joints, tendons, organs and the skin. When there is a disruption in this neuromuscular communication, the nervous system senses something is wrong and tells the body either through pain, autonomic signs like a change in blood pressure or through muscle weakness or spasm. AK helps to pinpoint this communication failure and alleviate it at its source. This alleviation from a successful therapeutic intervention results in an immediate and measurable improvement in the function of the muscle(s) being tested. FMT essentially measures whether a muscle is physiologically *facilitated* (functioning) or *inhibited* (not functioning). Its goal is to find the problematic muscle(s) and restore maximum functionality. In AK, this is known as *turning a muscle back on.*

How can *turning a muscle on* achieve such immediate results? Traditional wisdom states that it is not possible to increase muscle "strength" without weeks of exercise and proper nutrition. This is true, and herein lies the source of the confusion that some doctors (and patients) have with AK. Applied Kinesiologists are NOT changing muscle *strength*; they are changing muscle *function.* Muscle *strength* cannot be changed in the blink of an eye, but muscle *function* can because it relies on facilitating the neural impulses that regulate it. These impulses can be restored in real time because of what is called the *plasticity* of the nervous system.

Plasticity essentially means the body's neural system can adapt to stimuli, both internal and external. Once it senses that any particular part of the body's system needs to adapt, the process begins to address whatever condition that arises. However, if there is a fundamental blockage that prevents the nervous system from initiating the necessary change, it creates a dysfunction. FMT is able to locate the blockage and indicate the best therapeutic options to remove it so that the adaptive process can take its course and restore healthy function. This powerful diagnostic tool measures obstacles to natural plasticity—allowing the AK specialist to remove them and restore proper function.

How can a simple muscle test represent a window into factors beyond the dysfunctional muscle being tested? As stated earlier, one of the significant values of AK is as a diagnostic tool for an individual's total health. The homeostasis of the body depends on the interrelationship of its muscular-skeletal-endocrine systems. The vast network of muscles and tissues that surround the skeletal bones or skeletal muscles comprise one of the largest organ systems in the body. They secrete small but important proteins, known as *myokines,* that have a variety of functions. Principal among these functions is that they facilitate the signaling between muscles, organs and the general nervous system. Myokines are released into circulation during exercise and are thought to protect against a group of diseases including type 2 diabetes, cardiovascular disease, cancer, dementia, and osteoporosis.[8,9] When a condition exists that blocks this signaling, it often manifests in muscle dysfunction which can become a source of pain and affect the overall health and mobility of a person. Therefore, muscle dysfunction revealed through muscle testing may be due to a signal it is receiving, or not receiving, from a different part of the body. Once diagnosed, a trained AK professional can "unblock" the signaling process by restoring normal muscle function and relieve the impact on the body in general.

As miraculous as AK can be, it has its limits. AK does not treat pathological conditions such as fractures, cancer, tumors, and other chronic conditions. AK deals with the functional and fixable causes that are often overlooked or misdiagnosed by traditional medical procedures. Even so, in selected cases of pathology, AK treatments can most certainly help to ameliorate some pain and discomfort and can help the body to function at as high a level as possible in the context of the disease. Often, it might help to prevent certain conditions from getting worse.

However, at its core, AK represents a more proactive approach to health than a reactive response to disease.

Examination, Diagnosis, and Treatment

Applied Kinesiology is first and foremost a diagnostic discipline. As such, there is a detailed procedure to follow before the AK professional can discover the nature of your problem. It begins with a questionnaire. Most of us are used to filling out some kind of medical profile when visiting a physician for the first time. It contains the usual personal information, questions about medical history, medications and some questions regarding lifestyle. While it provides a medical context for the health profile of a patient, it doesn't give the physician much by way of diagnostic information.

The initial AK medical profile is much more extensive. It contains additional standard questions about a person's medical history, list of medications and allergies. A typical profile starts with the patient answering nearly 200 questions about an array of symptoms you may or may not be experiencing by checking one of three boxes concerning severity: mild, moderate or severe. The patient lists five main health concerns at the time of the visit as well as the reason for the appointment.

One of the more unique elements in an AK profile is that it asks the patient to draw a schematic diagram of any area of pain or discomfort. The diagram is annotated, using letters to indicate the type and location of the patient's pain and sensations: A=ache; B=burning; S=stabbing; N= numbness; P=pins & needles; O=other. Lastly, the patient describes the level of pain in each location from 0 (no pain) to 10 (severe pain).

Once your profile is complete, you are ready for your examination. An Applied Kinesiologist begins the examination the moment he or she sees you move. All movement is a function of your muscles, and every move you make is an important indicator of how the body is adapting to the condition. As you stand up, as you extend your hand, as you breathe, as you walk, even as you make every facial expression—a trained Applied Kinesiologist is well versed in understanding your body language to uncover health issues and is observing every aspect of muscle function as he or she begins to form a diagnosis.

When you stand from the chair, an Applied Kinesiologist is watching to see if your gluteal muscles in your hips and the quadriceps muscles in your thighs are functioning to help you to rise up in a smooth, balanced glide or if you are you shifting to one side or even using your arms to lift yourself out of the chair. If you have trouble straightening up, then perhaps the main hip flexors, the psoas muscles, are tight and not allowing you to stand up straight for the first five steps or so.

When you extend your hand to shake the doctor's hand, is the shoulder rising up due to pain or restriction in the neck area? Is there a lack of freedom in the elbow or shoulder? Is the grip of the handshake as strong as it should be, or is there possible nerve impingement in the neck, thoracic/chest area, shoulder, elbow or possibly a carpal tunnel syndrome?

We breathe approximately 20,000 times a day. As we breathe normally, the ribcage expands filling our lungs with air. Are the neck muscles straining or nostrils flaring, exhibiting some difficulty in the lungs filling completely with each breath? Are the abdominals relaxing and then contracting so your ribs can freely open and close like an oxygen-mobilizing accordion? Is there any shortness of breath?

Facial muscles reveal the level of pain or discomfort of a patient as well as one's general emotional state. Your facial movements show how the cranial bones and nerves are functioning. When you speak, the way you move (or don't move) your mouth can reveal if there is tightness in your facial muscles and how much tension is in one of the most important joints in the body, the jaw or the temporomandibular joint (TMJ).

As you walk down the hall to the consultation room, the doctor will watch how you carry yourself commonly known as your gait. *Gait Analysis* is the first general diagnostic tool. Based on the trained eye of the AK professional, he or she can learn an incredible amount by observing how a patient walks. The length of the stride can indicate some muscle weakness with your hip flexor or quadriceps muscle in the front of your thigh or tightness in the hamstrings in the back of your thigh. If the patient leans to one side, it may indicate an issue with a specific muscle in the lower back. If your feet flare out while walking, it might point to a weakness in the knee. If the arms don't move in tandem while walking, it might indicate some issue with the spine and shoulder blades.

During the consultation, your doctor will ask you a series of questions based on the detailed medical profile you've completed that directly relate to the reason for the visit. It is vital for him or her to hear you describe your concerns in your own words. Patients will often give clues to dysfunction with certain phrases such as, "I am so nervous all the time" or "I feel screwed up" or "I feel like it's all in my head." Common assessments such as these alert your doctor to a wide variety of possible conditions that may need to be examined further. Applied Kinesiology teaches doctors that if they listen carefully, the patient will give clues as to the actual source of their problem.

The consultation is basically the time where your doctor is looking for these clues to help solve your health problem. These clues do not only come from what the patient is saying. A trained Applied Kinesiologist is listening intently and also continues to observe your every movement, particularly hand movements. Patients will often unconsciously touch an area that they do not even realize is connected to the problem. More often than not, they might touch an area that is not part of the discussion, which could indicate another problem as well.

After the consultation, the AK specialist will review any X-rays, MRIs, CAT scans and blood work you may have brought with you. These provide valuable information and also serve to rule out conditions that may require surgery or other medical procedures.

After the general consultation, the examination continues with standard orthopedic and neurological tests as well as your vital signs such as blood pressure, pulse, respiratory rate, and temperature. An Applied Kinesiologist will often take multiple blood pressures with you sitting, standing and lying down. Changes in blood pressure in these different positions can reveal a health issue with your kidneys or adrenal glands.

Your exam then moves on to *Postural Analysis*, which gives your Applied Kinesiologist general information about how one's muscles function when standing. Postural distortions such as an uneven shoulder height or curvature of the spine often indicate a muscle problem that needs to be fixed.

Your doctor then will move on to *Temporal/Sphenoidal Line Analysis* (TS Line). This is a procedure whereby you lie face up on the examination table, and your Applied Kinesiologist will manually evaluate the temporalis muscle. The temporalis muscle is the largest muscle of the jaw that fans out on both sides of your head. Tightness here is a common cause of headaches, and tender points in this muscle can serve as an indication of problems elsewhere in the body.

Finally, there is *Acupuncture Pulse Point Analysis*. This analysis is based on the 5000-year-old science of classical acupuncture. It has identified a series of energetic pathways throughout the body known as meridians. There are various points over the radial artery on the inside of your wrists that can clue the clinician into where there is a blockage or excess of energy flowing through the meridians. As you place your fingers in three locations over your radial arteries located near both wrists, the Applied Kinesiologist will use specific muscle testing to see if there is a problem with your meridians. If a blockage is found, the doctor will note it as the examination continues. Later, he or she may gently engage acupressure points along with spinal adjustments and herbs to restore homeostasis to this important energetic system flowing in your body.

After assembling this information, the AK professional is now prepared to employ the fundamental diagnostic tool of AK—FMT.

Muscle testing is the final part of the examination that will lead to a comprehensive diagnosis and treatment plan. Your doctor will begin by focusing on those muscles that appeared to be most problematic when you move, walk and stand as well as those revealed in your temporalis muscle (TS Line) and your acupuncture system. Muscle testing takes the guesswork out of the equation and lets the Applied Kinesiologist know if you have a functional problem and how it can best be treated.

If the tests indicate a purely functional issue, your doctor will discuss it with you and describe the treatment plan. Once an Applied Kinesiologist finds the source of your problem, he or she will treat it until normal function is restored. Depending upon the severity of the specific condition along with the general health status of the individual, successful resolution may take a few simple procedures on the first visit, or it may take several visits, weeks, or even months. Each person's body will respond differently. In the vast majority of cases, however, the condition will be alleviated completely in a short period. Of equal importance, your AK practitioner will teach you what to do to prevent the condition from recurring through specific exercises, nutritional supplements, and lifestyle changes. This patient education process is paramount to the successful restoration and attainment of true optimal health. In the unlikely event that the condition is not totally functional in nature, the AK specialist will suggest that you consult a specialist to address any nonfunctional concerns.

Albert Einstein said, "Nothing happens until something moves." While this simple statement referred to the world of theoretical physics, it seems prescient with regards to AK. One of its basic tenants is that *movement is medicine*. Since you need to move every day, you also need to make sure your muscles are functioning and that your joints are in proper alignment if you want to enjoy optimal health and be pain-free. That is the principal goal of AK—to heal dysfunction and prevent it from recurring.

AK trains doctors to treat the *person* with the condition; not the *condition* experienced by the person. Functional muscle testing coordinates the pieces of the diagnostic puzzle to assess the complete person. It is for this reason that people turn to an AK professional. His or her holistic and individualized methodology of treating the inner cause and not the outer effect is the great contribution of AK to medicine and the healing arts.

3

APPLIED KINESIOLOGY AND OTHER HEALING DISCIPLINES

AK began as an extension of the chiropractic discipline and derives much of its diagnostic and treatment focus on its fundamental concept of the healthy alignment of the body's complex structure. Through the use of precise observation of a person's movements and the unique method of functional manual muscle testing, a trained AK specialist can pinpoint the source of a patient's complaint and create a treatment plan that will restore him or her to optimal health. In many cases, if the principal source of the problem is muscular dysfunction, an AK professional can get the muscle functioning properly again by specific muscle manipulation, followed by precise adjustments to the underlying skeletal structure.

However, it doesn't stop there. What makes AK so powerful it that its fundamental perspective reflects the nature of the body itself. The body is a complicated and fully integrated collection of systems all working in tandem to maintain its overall homeostasis. Each of these systems operates according to its function in the body and is interconnected with the others through the neurons that modulate them. If one system is not working optimally, it can affect many others and upset the body's natural balance, which leads to disease or other lapses in the health of an individual.

AK has reverence for this model and is one of the few healing disciplines that respects and incorporates the best of a wide variety of other healing disciplines to achieve optimal health. This integrative model stands in stark contrast to the fragmented approach of traditional medicine in which a patient visits a series of specialists, each with their own diagnosis as it relates to their specialty, often with little to no coordination with others. What can emerge is a maze of information, which often leads to a grab bag of medications and procedures that do little to treat the entire patient effectively. Think of an orchestra comprised of virtuoso performers, each playing their own part without the insights and guidance of a conductor. The end result is chaos.

The great benefit of AK is that it provides a path to healing that utilizes the deep knowledge of other medical professions and disciplines. Due to its integrative perspective, it aggregates all the information concerning the patient's medical profile and general lifestyle through its individualized examination process to create a clear diagnosis and treatment plan. Often the AK practitioner can treat the patient using a wide variety of disciplines. However, if the patient's diagnosis involves a pathological condition, the AK professional will do what he or she can to ameliorate the symptoms before, during and after the intervention by another medical professional.

Applied Kinesiology and Chiropractic

Applied Kinesiology is based upon the chiropractic premise that "structure determines function." Therefore, when the structures of the body are out of alignment, they don't function properly—often leading to painful conditions. People wishing to avoid pain start moving less, and a vicious cycle is perpetuated leading to weight gain, arthritis, nerve entrapment, and general ill health resulting in more pain.

Applied Kinesiology enhances this chiropractic principle of proper joint motion by promoting proper function to the muscles surrounding each joint. Precise alignments to joints will not hold if the muscles that are designed to keep them in place are malfunctioning—being either too weak or too tight. Applied Kinesiology's manual muscle manipulation can facilitate functionality of these muscles and ensure the lasting health benefits of proper alignments.

APPLIED KINESIOLOGY AND PHYSICAL THERAPY

The connection between AK and physical therapy (PT) is an important and vastly overlooked one. Applied Kinesiology and physical therapy are, by their nature, synergistic. PT and rehabilitation are essential to mitigating the effects of an injury or chronic muscular condition to restore injured muscles to full functionality and strength. While it is vital that an individual with these issues undergo a program of strengthening and rehabilitation, few realize that their muscles need to be prepared before the program begins. Just as with chiropractic adjustments, unless the muscles are *physiologically* functioning properly, they won't derive the full benefit from PT.

Applied Kinesiology's proven techniques are essential to the total healing process and should be implemented before a comprehensive PT regimen is started. In other words, for optimal results from rehabilitative exercises—*physiological* therapy (AK) should precede *physical* therapy (PT). Therefore, injured muscles need to be *physiologically strengthened* by AK procedures and then *physically strengthened* by PT exercises.

APPLIED KINESIOLOGY AND ACUPUNCTURE

Fundamental to the ancient science of acupuncture is its use of the complex energy pathways through the body known as *meridians.* These pathways serve to keep the muscles and other organs operating in perfect balance. AK recognizes that precise attention to an imbalance or blockage in these meridians can be instrumental in restoring muscle function. The skilled Applied Kinesiologist can treat most cases of meridian imbalance with special techniques without the use of needles such as the Pain Gate Control Technique that has been clinically proven to be highly effective in ameliorating pain naturally.[10] The procedure involves the doctor using Acupuncture Pulse Point Analysis to diagnose which one of the approximately 365 acupuncture points is most associated with the pain of the individual patient and tapping it gently for two minutes. The tapping stimulates specific receptors known as mechanoreceptors; this stimulation blocks the receptors known as nociceptors from carrying signals up the spinal cord to be perceived as pain in the brain.

However, if muscle testing shows a reoccurring issue, or if symptoms persist that are most likely due to a pervasive meridian imbalance, the Applied Kinesiologist will refer the patient to an acupuncturist.

Applied Kinesiology and Dentistry

Many people are surprised to learn that dental patients can benefit from specific AK techniques. The jaw, also known as the temporomandibular joint (TMJ), is among the most active joints in the body, moving about 2,000 times daily.[11] Studies have shown that 35-40% of brain function is manifested through the face and head. Accordingly, problems involving the TMJ can have a widespread impact on the general muscular-skeletal system. One example is that dysfunction in the TMJ is linked to painful spinal curvature conditions known as scoliosis.

Functional manual muscle testing is often used to determine if a patient's occlusion (bite) is causing tension in the jaw, head, and neck. For example, TMJ disorders have clinically been found to be a common cause of *bruxism* (teeth grinding), *tinnitus* (ear ringing) and jaw clicking. There is also some evidence that the tremendously painful facial condition known as *trigeminal neuralgia* can be relieved by a TMJ correction. Additionally, TMJ dysfunction is associated with lower back pain as well as cold hands and feet.

If your jaw muscles are found to be *hypertonic* (too tense), AK muscle manipulation techniques to the neuromuscular spindle cells along with therapy to the fascia of the jaw muscles will relieve the tension in the TMJ. An Applied Kinesiologist is able to expertly determine which position of the jaw is causing the most tension and is able to relieve the muscular imbalance and restore the alignment to this delicate joint.

After making these muscular corrections, the AK professional will recommend that your dentist fit you for a bite-correcting appliance to help the TMJ remain in place. When the dentist rectifies the malocclusion and restores an optimal bite position, muscle testing will confirm the success of the procedure, and patients will find relief from any symptoms he or she experienced from this issue.

Applied Kinesiology and Traditional Medicine

While there is a fundamental difference between the approach to healing of traditional medicine and AK, professionals in each discipline can derive great benefits from working together for the optimal health of patients. Ideally, if medical doctors or specialists were trained in the diagnostic and curative techniques of AK, they could address the complaints of many of the people they treat more effectively.

Cardiologists using functional muscle manipulation testing procedures could identify and treat myofascial trigger points of the pectoral muscles, which can cause pain erroneously attributed to *myocardial infarction*—more commonly known as a heart attack. Using these techniques can also help in the prescription of nutritional supplements that support healthy heart function such as vitamins B and E, coenzyme Q10, acetyl-L-carnitine, and magnesium, to name a few.

Gastroenterologists could use AK to ensure that the *psoas* and *abdominal* muscles are functioning properly. The *psoas* muscle has connections with the fascial covering of the intestines (peritoneum) and aids in keeping them in proper position within the abdominal cavity to support the other digestive organs. Malfunction can lead to a condition known as ptosis, wherein an organ drops down or breaks through the abdominal wall. Hernias are one example of this problem.

The psoas connection includes a close relationship to the ileocecal valve that lies between the small and large intestine and can disrupt its important function of ensuring that waste meant to leave your body through the large intestine does not seep back into the small intestine to be absorbed into the bloodstream. The psoas also connects to the diaphragm, and an imbalance in the tone, function or strength of either psoas muscle might lead to acid reflux and/or a hiatal hernia, where the stomach slides up into the chest cavity. Traditional medicine is aware of the connection of the psoas with the intestines and has a standard medical test called the *psoas sign* which, along with other signs and symptoms, can be an indication of appendicitis (inflammation of the appendix). Such a sign occurs if hyperextension or contraction of the hip causes friction against nearby inflamed tissues, since the psoas muscle borders the peritoneal cavity. AK functional muscle testing represents a refinement of this basic use of the psoas muscle for diagnosis.

There is an AK technique whereby the doctor manipulates the ileocecal valve (ICV) to relieve any possible spasms. The procedure entails a directional manipulation of the intestine to mechanically correct any dysfunction of the valve, which is muscular in nature. Due to an unwanted backflow of toxic waste into the body, Applied Kinesiologists have found ICV disturbances to be a frequent cause of a wide range of maladies including severe low back pain, headaches, fatigue, menstrual problems, and even bad breath. Regarding the digestive tract, this technique has proven to be of great help in patients with constipation or diarrhea of unknown origin, as well as cases of irritable bowel, bloating and diverticulitis. It can help gastroenterologists find a functional cause for their patient's distress.

Under our current medical system, the institutions that train doctors have yet to recognize the power of AK as a tool of deep and lasting healing. As the awareness of AK as a legitimate medical discipline grows, the medical profession may be best served to incorporate it as part of the training for all medical practitioners. At present, forward-thinking medical professionals who value a more holistic approach to treatment must take the initiative to participate in the training on their own.

Applied Kinesiology and Psychotherapy

Psychotherapy benefits from utilizing several techniques unique to AK concerning conditions related to the emotional health of patients. These procedures are an adjunct to traditional psychotherapy and represent physical interventions that can have an immediate effect on the psychological state of an individual. Generally speaking, some involve gentle manipulation of specific receptors on the forehead; others involve tapping acupuncture points during moments of stress; another is a form of self-hypnosis you can do while stimulating the temporal area of your head.

Many of these techniques are clinically effective in helping people with anxiety, self-sabotaging behaviors, and physical effects from unresolved emotional stress, as well as in supporting athletic and academic performance and weight loss programs. Any certified Applied Kinesiologist can apply these techniques and can also teach the patient how to implement versions of them at home to relieve the physical aspects of an emotional condition. However, AK techniques must work in conjunction with a psychotherapist to address any psychological source of the problem.

This dual approach of incorporating physical and psychological therapeutic modalities is important because there are two major categories of dysfunction in the mind/body connection: *psychosomatic* and *somatopsychic. Psychosomatic* dysfunction is a commonly misunderstood term connoting a condition involving physical problems that exist only in the imagination of the patient. However, this condition is all too real. The mind can affect the body, particularly as related to emotional stress. Examples of stress-related physical manifestations include hypertension, rashes, pain, and Takotsubo cardiomyopathy—also known as *acute stress-induced cardiomyopathy* or "broken-heart syndrome."

Somatopsychic dysfunction is the reverse. It occurs when a physiological condition causes an emotional or psychological reaction. Common examples include temper outbursts brought on by low blood sugar, mental confusion as a consequence of tight jaw and facial muscles causing a restriction of the cranial bones, and depression due to a B12 deficiency—which is prevalent among people over the age of 50 and among vegetarians. Applied Kinesiologists have noted that nearly any physical problem can create or contribute to accompanying emotional symptoms.

Acupuncture science attributes this body/mind relationship to blockages in the energy meridians associated with specific emotional states such as depression, anxiety, fear, anger, and elation.

Acupuncture therapy, along with manual muscle manipulation and testing, has proven successful in treating these emotional symptoms.

Applied Kinesiology specialists have empirically observed "emotional releases" after the application of AK physical therapeutic interventions. For instance, patients will inexplicably laugh, cry, or remember past traumas previously unavailable to them after a deep fascial manipulation of chronically tight muscles—which in all likelihood were tight and painful due to the very same stress these individuals are emotionally recalling and releasing. Patients might become panic-stricken with objective signs of elevated pulse rate, blushing, and profuse sweating when they think about speaking in public or getting on an airplane. Then, within a minute of the doctor treating the "Emotional Recall Receptors" on the forehead, the very same visceral reactions dissipate, and the patient is now calm when thinking about the exact same *previously terrifying* scenarios.

These techniques measure the effects of the patient's mental/emotional status on the neuromuscular system and show how treating the body can correctly dampen this vicious cycle, which may have started within the psyche. AK has been able to develop physical techniques to more specifically and effectively bring these emotional releases about in a more controlled way and restore the body to homeostasis.

The success of these AK techniques to help patients with emotional stress, phobia-like symptoms, and "performance anxiety" syndromes has led to creating a burgeoning field known as *Energy Psychology*. From the groundbreaking work of AK there have developed various schools of *Energy Psychology,* such as Thought Field Therapy (TFT), Neuro Emotional Technique (NET), and Emotional Freedom Technique (EFT). TFT, NET, and EFT rely on tapping reflex points within the acupuncture system (NET also adds specific spinal adjustments to influence the nervous system) while asserting positive affirmations and/or observing the effects of certain memories or thoughts upon the neuromuscular system. These represent unique techniques derived from AK fundamentals that address the health issue from a functional vantage point.

Eye Movement Desensitization and Reprocessing (EMDR) is another technique closely associated with the basic AK concept that "movement is medicine." A psychologist reportedly discovered EMDR independently, and studies have found it to be effective in certain cases of posttraumatic stress disorder (PTSD). Even though EMDR does not claim to be derived from AK, its protocol is very similar, and it has been readily implemented into certain AK procedures.

There is a timeless saying that, "If the only tool you have is a hammer, everything looks like a nail." This means that if a person relies on only one way of doing something, he will approach issues from that single perspective. What makes AK truly and uniquely powerful is that it accepts information from all health modalities without prejudice. This respect for the potential contributions from such a wide range of sources ensures a patient the most comprehensive treatment plan available to restore true health.

4

THE TRIAD OF HEALTH

As we've seen, AK treats the whole person, not just the symptoms he or she might present with. Its goal is to restore and maintain the total health and homeostasis of the individual seeking treatment. The fundamental concept that exemplifies this goal is *The Triad of Health*. It recognizes three basic factors that influence wellness: the physiological/physical, the nutritional/chemical, and the psychological/emotional. The relationship between these important elements of well-being is constantly changing. Maintaining balance among these three factors will keep you on your journey to good and lasting health. AK is one of the only healing disciplines to recognize the importance of this Triad of Health, especially as it affects the interaction between the nervous system and the organs and muscles.

Currently, traditional health care uses an essentially piecemeal approach to addressing your health issues. When a condition presents itself, the patient needs to navigate a path between medical specialists with different, and sometimes confusingly different, approaches. Quite often there are conflicting diagnoses and treatments, and the patient is left bewildered and still suffering from the condition.

AK looks at the larger canvas of healing by promoting the balance of the three essential parts of the Triad of Health. By paying attention to your physical health through healthy exercise, getting enough sleep and regular chiropractic adjustments, you will help to ensure that your muscles, bones, and joints will remain strong. Nourish yourself through a nutritious diet and supplements, avoiding toxins in foods filled with artificial chemicals, and drink purified water. Try to avoid unnecessary stress and exposure to destructive emotional situations and nurture your mind and spirit with meditation or some other calming technique to keep your psyche in balance. These efforts will help prevent dysfunction.

However, our best efforts to support the Triad of Health often can't prevent health problems entirely. When you are not feeling your best, experiencing pain and/or some other condition, there is usually some imbalance present. Often, this imbalance is difficult to find. Through AK's diagnostic methods, a trained professional will pinpoint the imbalance and create a clear path to the best way to treat it.

How does your Applied Kinesiologist discover which of the three factors is out of balance? Regarding the physical, he or she relies upon the detailed information from the patient and any medical tests that he or she might have undergone. As part of the diagnostic regimen, there is also a technique unique to AK that serves as a window into a patient's health, known as Therapy Localization (TL).

In 1974, Dr. Goodheart reported that when a patient placed his or her hand over a problem area, there was a change in the result of the functional manual muscle test. Following this shift, it enabled him to ascertain the location where treatment needed to be applied. In many cases, the underlying dysfunction was not located in the area indicated by the patient but in another part of his or her body. Goodheart dubbed this phenomenon—Therapy Localization.

The underlying premise of TL is that the body is holographic in nature. As in a hologram or three-dimensional image, all the properties and information of the subject are integrated throughout the image. No matter where you look, the basic qualities of the image remain the same. Similarly, every system and part of the human body is interrelated and remains in constant connection. Therefore, a disruption in one area of the body can lead to an understanding of what is affecting it as a physiological whole.

TL has advanced since its discovery in 1974. While it began by having the patient place his or her hand over the area believed to be the source of the imbalance, the technique has now been expanded to having the AK professional instruct the patient to contact and apply pressure to various parts of the body to locate multiple contributing factors to the patient's problems. Recent studies have proven the efficacy of TL as a powerful tool that any doctor trained in AK can implement into his or her practice to discover where the imbalance in the patient's physiology is and how best to treat the root cause of that individual's problem.[12,13]

Nutrition is vitally important to maintain the balance of the Triad of Health. In conjunction with traditional blood and urine tests, AK also uses the body's sense of taste to discover nutritional imbalances. When we taste something, the sensation is immediately transmitted from our taste buds located in the tongue directly to your brain.

Once the neurological message of taste is registered in your brain, it is simultaneously sent through your spinal cord to the alpha motor neurons that affect your muscles and to your autonomic nervous system. Changes in muscle function occur in response to the particular taste experience, which may indicate an imbalance in nutrition. Once discovered through precise muscle testing, the AK professional can prescribe the appropriate supplements and dietary changes to restore the balance.

For example, Applied Kinesiologists routinely test for a magnesium deficiency. In addition to supporting over 700 enzymes in the body, magnesium is important for muscle function and in relieving muscle spasms—including those of the heart. It also helps with increasing blood vessel elasticity. A magnesium deficiency has been shown to lead to persistent muscle dysfunction, as well as cardiovascular diseases such as mitral valve prolapses, irregular heartbeat (arrhythmia), hypertrophic cardiomyopathy, angina, and heart attacks.

Through years of research and testing, AK has shown the correlation between a specific shoulder muscle, the *subscapularis* and heart issues. Because this shoulder muscle is used extensively by athletes, it becomes a primary focus of an AK specialist in these patients. If the subscapularis displays inhibited function, the doctor will have the patient taste a magnesium supplement and observe if there is a positive response in the functional manual muscle test. If so, the doctor will recommend this nutritional supplement as well as foods that are rich sources of magnesium such as spinach, broccoli, almonds, pumpkin seeds, raisins, bananas, and dark chocolate to support the physical treatment program.

Stress, which is basically a syndrome of heightened awareness of an individual to a wide variety of experiences, is the most common disruptor of the emotional/psychological component of the Triad of Health. The American Association of Family Physicians reports that approximately two-thirds of all doctor visits are due to stress-related ailments.[14] AK's unique ability to use functional muscle testing as a neural feedback mechanism to measure nervous system activity, and its immediate effect on the neuromuscular system allows your doctor to discover whether psychological stress is contributing to your health issues.

Small levels of stress can actually help us by giving us more energy to achieve our goals. However, when we surpass our individual stress tolerance threshold, there is an imbalance in the psycho-emotional aspect of the Triad.

Simply thinking about a stressful situation can cause changes throughout your entire body such as raising your blood pressure and pulse rate, increasing sweat gland activity, and causing an inhibition or tightening of your muscles. Your Applied Kinesiologist can detect these changes—much like a polygraph does in screening for lies.

For instance, stomach conditions such as acid reflux, ulcers, gastritis, and even simple nausea or nervous *butterflies* are often associated with stress. The muscle most closely associated with your stomach is the *pectoralis major clavicular* (PMC). Your AK professional will ask you to visualize or "think about" the particular situation that is causing stress. Using FMT, the AK professional will see if the PMC becomes physiologically inhibited during this visualization process. If this visualization causes a negative reaction and your muscle becomes inhibited, your doctor will investigate to see if certain stress-reducing techniques can mitigate its detrimental effects on your body.

A common "stress receptor" technique used in AK to relieve the stress impacting a person's health is known as Emotional Recall Technique (ERT). In this simple procedure, your doctor gently contacts the *stress receptors* on your forehead while you bring into your consciousness specific events, past or present, that are causing you duress. The receptors are held until your body displays physical signs of relief such as more relaxed breathing, facial serenity, lowering of pulse and blood pressure, and a decrease in muscle dysfunction. This technique relieves stress-related stomach conditions and also facilitates relaxation throughout your entire body—often giving relief from stress-induced headaches, backaches, and overall anxiety.

There are other techniques your Applied Kinesiologist can utilize such as Neurological Disorganization Syndrome Correction (which addresses ADHD and learning disabilities), Psychological Reversal Technique (common in self-sabotaging behaviors and in performance anxiety), Temporal Tapping (self-hypnosis), Injury Recall Technique (to relieve stress caused by residual physiological effects of a trauma), and the Anxiety Release Technique (sometimes called, The Five-Minute Phobia Cure.).

While ERT is the most basic of these powerful stress-relieving procedures, it represents the foundational emotional technique to help restore homeostasis to this piece of the Triad of Health. Relieving physical manifestations of stress allows a patient to concentrate on addressing the psychological component more effectively. Psychotherapy is always recommended in conjunction with these AK procedures.

AK is a functional treatment modality that employs specific techniques to help your body restore balance in the Triad of Health. However, *maintaining* the balance of the three elements in the Triad is the principal way to keep you on the journey to health. Many people will focus on one aspect, such as exercise, diet or meditation, unaware that it is the assimilation of all three that ultimately dictates your health. The interactions of these three major factors are constantly shifting.

AK takes into account that different aspects of the Triad are in play daily and will address whatever factor is most prevalent with regards to any current dysfunction. Each person is unique, and the simple fact is that your health is the sum total of the interactions between the physical, the nutritional and the emotional aspects of the Triad of Health. AK is able to deduce which of these various factors are the true causes that create your health difficulties—which are as unique for you as your fingerprint.

PART II

TREATING PEOPLE WITH VARIOUS CONDITIONS

5

SHOULDER AND ARM CONDITIONS

The shoulder is actually a complex of joints and has the most diverse and greatest range of motion of any area in the body. Utilizing more than twenty different muscles, the shoulder's varied range of movements allows us to perform a wide range of activities such as swimming, playing tennis, gardening, rowing a boat, and all forms of manual activities. Its main function is to give strength and mobility to the arm. However, the shoulder is also one of the most unstable and frequently injured areas of the body.

Four main joints comprise the shoulder complex. The first is the glenohumeral (GH) joint, which is a large ball and socket joint where the "rotator cuff" muscles attach. The GH is the most mobile joint in your body and is the most frequently dislocated joint in the body. The second joint is the acromioclavicular (AC), where your collarbone loosely connects to the shoulder blade. The third joint is the sternoclavicular (SC), where the other end of your collarbone attaches to the ribcage or, more specifically, your breastbone. The fourth joint is the scapulothoracic (ST), where the shoulder blade connects to the ribcage. The ST is known as a "physiological joint" because, while it has functional movement, there is no true bone-to-bone connection—technically the definition of a joint.

Many shoulder and arm issues are due to trauma usually from sports or strenuous activities such as weightlifting. Even so-called "safe" exercises, such as stretching, yoga, and Pilates, can be common causes of shoulder injuries if not done correctly. Shoulder problems can also occur gradually, often initiated by such routine tasks as lifting a package or a child incorrectly. Unless they are acute, we tend to attribute the annoying aches and pains to simply getting older and we "just learn to live with them." In most cases, there is no need to live with shoulder and arm pain. AK offers many solutions that enable patients to live pain-free and maintain their mobility.

When diagnosing shoulder conditions, medical professionals will use the terms bursitis, tendonitis, or arthritis. These terms are generic categories of conditions that don't really give you a detailed sense of what the true cause of your shoulder pain is and leads to a series of limited treatments such as anti-inflammatories, physical therapy exercises, ice, heat and cortisone shots. While these might alleviate discomfort temporarily, they don't treat the actual cause of the condition. AK delves deeper into the multitude of factors that contribute to and exacerbate any shoulder condition to find the cause and cure it permanently. These potential causes include poor biomechanics (especially posture), stress, daily physical activities, and dangerous exercise habits—along with common traumatic injuries.

Conditions Associated with Shoulder Pain and Arm Weakness

DONNA, 35, was living with severe, sharp pain in the front of her right shoulder for several weeks. She went to her general practitioner who diagnosed her pain as bursitis. He prescribed the anti-inflammatory ibuprofen, commonly known under the brand name Advil®. It helped a little, but Donna knew it was not getting to the cause of her pain and did not want to "live on Advil® forever" due to its accumulative negative health effects, including liver damage. A friend referred her to a chiropractor. The chiropractor also diagnosed her with bursitis and treated it with ultrasound and gave her a few standard exercises. She enjoyed greater relief in that she no longer felt the pain constantly. However, whenever she tried to exercise, the sharp pain would return immediately and prevent her from continuing.

The chiropractor saw that he was not getting to the root cause and referred her to another chiropractor who was also an Applied Kinesiologist. During the initial patient interview, Donna explained that the sharp pain first occurred when she was lifting her daughter's dance bag out of her truck. Now the pain came "out of nowhere" and struck most notably when she tried to perform pushups and whenever she carried laundry, groceries, or the infamous dance bag. Donna also related that she had difficulty in placing her hand into her front pants pocket.

The Applied Kinesiologist asked her to pinpoint the pain. Donna pointed to a distinct area on the front of her shoulder. When the doctor gently pressed on the area, it felt like a taut rubber band. Donna cried out in pain. The doctor had her stand (Postural Analysis) and then walk down the hallway (Gait Analysis). In both instances, it was apparent that Donna kept her right arm significantly straighter than her left and that her right shoulder was positioned slightly more forward.

As the examination continued, the doctor asked her to sit on the examination table and raise her arm. Donna reported that she had sharp pain while initially raising the arm. However, when the elbow went past the horizontal position to her body, she was then able to proceed with very little pain. This sign of pain diminishing once the arm went past the horizontal, plus the location of the sharp pain, led the Applied Kinesiologist to suspect that Donna's problem stemmed from a biceps tendon that may have slipped out of position and became compromised.

The doctor then continued with the examination by using AK FMT. The biceps muscle was weak and painful to contract. Since one function of the biceps is to stabilize the shoulder and another is to flex (bend) the elbow, this would explain why Donna's right shoulder was slightly ahead of her left and why she held her right arm conspicuously straighter than the other arm with the normally functioning biceps.

Using TL, the doctor tested the muscle again while Donna placed her hand over the shoulder, specifically over the biceps tendon. While Donna maintained this hand contact over the biceps tendon, the biceps muscle became strong (physiologically facilitated) and did not hurt when she flexed it.

Then the doctor employed a diagnostic technique that is unique to AK known as a Static Challenge. Its principal purpose is to evaluate the impact of a part of the body that may be out of alignment with muscles dependent upon it. The procedure is as follows: the doctor or patient holds a part of the body suspected of being out of alignment into the anatomically correct position while testing a specific muscle or set of muscles. If the muscle(s) becomes facilitated, it confirms the misalignment.

In this case, the doctor asked Donna to gently push the biceps tendon slightly inwards and then outwards. When Donna held the tendon in the inward direction, the biceps returned to its weakened and painful state. When she held the tendon in the outwards direction, the muscle regained its normal function and was no longer painful to contract.

Based on the examination, the initial diagnosis was bicipital tendonitis due to a slipped bicipital tendon. Generally, this condition is due to trauma while the biceps is flexed, usually after a sudden movement while carrying some heavy object. It is one of the most common causes of referral pain to the shoulder. This diagnosis fit Donna's experience perfectly.

Armed with a precise diagnosis, the treatment procedure involved slipping the tendon back into place. Donna sat where full motion of the arm could be realized. The doctor stabilized her forearm while the elbow was flexed to 90° and applied continual pressure using his thumb while gently pulling the arm down and backward. Then the doctor slowly brought the arm out to the side and rotated it while maintaining digital pressure on the tendon. As the arm was brought back to its starting position, there was an audible "click." This signified that the manipulation was successful, and the tendon had been restored to its proper position in the shoulder.

Once the tendon is back in place, *fascial release* is required to restore the normal length of the tendon, which automatically becomes shortened when out of position. This medical massage technique is used to restore normalcy to the fascia (connective tissue) that covers the entire biceps muscle. The fascia frequently tightens up due to abnormal tension while the tendon is out of place. Donna was instructed not to raise her arm over her head for three to seven days after treatment to prevent the tendon from slipping out of position. Use of ice over the area and anti-inflammatory nutrients or over-the-counter medications were recommended, as well as supplements with such ligament-supporting nutrients as manganese to ensure a complete recovery.

As is often the case, the tendon needed to be realigned with several subsequent visits until the ligaments regained their normal resiliency and held it in place. Donna ultimately enjoyed a complete recovery.

* * *

MICHAEL, 23, was a chiropractic student who was experiencing a constant ache and weakness in his left arm and shoulder. The other interns and even the experienced clinicians at his school, while able to help ameliorate some of the intense pain, could not fully remedy the condition. The X-ray report did not reveal any noticeable problem; MRIs were not performed. One of the doctors referred him to a colleague trained in AK.

During the consultation, Michael related that the sharp pain started after he adjusted the lower back of a classmate. He had not warmed up as he had been taught before attempting to deliver a precise chiropractic adjustment and felt a searing pain in his shoulder immediately. Postural and Gait Analysis revealed that Michael stood and walked with his left arm essentially pinned to his side and that his left shoulder was drooping down dramatically lower than his right.

His physical examination revealed that he was able to move the arm relatively pain-free until he brought his arm up to the last 30° of elevation. At this point, he would feel a sharp pain in the shoulder and extreme weakness in the arm. When asked exactly where he was experiencing pain, the patient pointed to the end of his collarbone directly above his shoulder.

The doctor asked him to get into the same position he had assumed when delivering the chiropractic adjustment when his pain began. He did so and found he had no strength in his arm, as if it were "dead." Previous chiropractic treatments had improved the shoulder to the point where he only experienced the sharp pain when he raised his arm up over his head. However, the constant ache and weakness persisted and prevented him from attempting to deliver a chiropractic adjustment. This disability not only affected his performance in chiropractic technique class but also his future as a licensed doctor of chiropractic after graduation. The doctor asked if there were other activities that he felt this "dead arm" sensation. Michael said that if he tried to throw a ball, do bench presses, or even blow-dry his hair, his arm also went "dead."

Upon close examination of the X-rays that were taken at the clinic, the doctor noted that there was an almost imperceptible space between the collarbone and the shoulder blade in the AC joint. When the AC joint is compromised, it creates dysfunction in the normal shoulder mechanics and the two muscles that directly cross the joint—the upper trapezius and the middle deltoid. The condition of this joint is best seen on X-ray when two pictures are taken; one without the patient holding anything and one with the patient holding a ten-pound weight. If there is an injury of the joint, the space will be measurably increased while the patient is holding the weight. However, as this second X-ray is not usually prescribed, this injury is often missed.

After muscle testing, the doctor noted weakness in these two shoulder muscles. Since both muscles were inhibited, it was the significant factor causing Michael's pain and arm weakness. Using the Static Challenge, the doctor held the injured joint together, essentially bracing it in the proper position, and tested the two muscles again. There was significant improvement in function and a decrease in pain. This confirmed a diagnosis of an acromioclavicular joint sprain/strain.

The doctor performed a gentle chiropractic adjustment to the joint, taped the shoulder area to keep it in place and prescribed specific exercises along with instructions to maintain good posture when sitting and standing. It was important to note that slouching would cause, among many other things, a strain to the AC joint. Michael required seven additional treatment sessions to *physiologically facilitate (strengthen)* the muscles and stabilize the ligaments and went on to enjoy a full recovery.

* * *

LETITIA, 42, experienced a constant ache and weakness in her right arm and shoulder after "pulling all-nighters" studying for the Law School Admission Test. She had raised her three children, was healthy and never experienced this kind of pain before. Her husband was a prominent medical doctor who was in the process of becoming certified in AK. He could not get to the bottom of the problem, and he referred her to his instructor who was a Diplomate in Applied Kinesiology with many years of experience.

During the consultation, Letitia stated that she had no memory of any physical trauma. The dull ache and weakness in her arm started while studying for her exams. X-rays and MRIs revealed no fractures, tumors or other pathology aside from some diffuse inflammation in the area, possibly indicative of tendonitis.

On Postural Analysis, the patient displayed that her right shoulder was noticeably displaced down and forward. Gait Analysis revealed *a disconnect* between the movement of her right arm with the rest of her body. It was as if her right arm was not a part of the rest of her.

Using a hand Dynamometer, a standard medical device that measures hand strength, she displayed a significant weakness in grip strength in her right hand compared to the left—even though she was right-handed. When the doctor placed his hand on the outer part of the shoulder, Letitia reacted quickly in pain. In this case, sharp pain signified a precise area of strain that was, in all likelihood, contributing to the patient's problem.

The examination proceeded to the functional muscle-testing portion, and the doctor noted that one of the four of the rotator cuff muscles, the *supraspinatus* muscle, was physiologically inhibited. In fact, it was so weak that the patient had difficulty putting the arm up into position to be tested, and it hurt when she attempted to do so.

The doctor then tested the shoulder muscle again, this time holding the arm up as if Letitia had it in a sling, to take the weight off of the joint. While maintaining this upward pressure, the muscle tested as fully functional and without pain. This clue gave the doctor what he was looking for. He diagnosed her condition as a slight dislocation of the shoulder (GH) due to a physiological inhibition of one of the rotator cuff muscles, specifically the supraspinatus. Applied Kinesiologists have learned that a dysfunction of the supraspinatus muscle can cause the shoulder to become slightly dislocated.

But this was not the only factor that contributed to Letitia's condition. Unlike other muscles in the shoulder, the supraspinatus muscle has been proven to be affected by brain fatigue. This fatigue caused by intense mental activity, such as long periods of study, can physiologically inhibit its proper function as well.

The doctor used a simple shoulder alignment to correct the dislocation. Letitia experienced immediate relief. She was instructed to apply ice for twenty minutes six times a day for three days and was advised to take nutrients such as fish oils and B vitamins as well as gotu kola and ginkgo biloba—herbs that support brain function. The doctor suggested that she eat foods believed to be excellent for the brain such as fish, walnuts and egg yolks. Most importantly, he advised her to take frequent breaks in her study by standing up and vigorously "walking in place" to oxygenate her brain and stimulate the supraspinatus muscle. The doctor also instructed her to get more sleep.

Letitia followed the instructions, and a follow up visit revealed that her shoulder had remained in place. Letitia was pain-free, more relaxed, and aced the LSAT.

Rotator Cuff Injury

FRANK, 55, was a former major league baseball pitcher turned manager. Part of his duties involved pitching to his players during batting practice. However, over a period of ten years after becoming a manager, he began to experience excruciating pain in his throwing arm. At first, it was intermittent, and he just fluffed it off. However, it got so bad that he went to the team doctors who diagnosed him with a rotator cuff condition and treated him for the pain with ibuprofen, cortisone shots, and a series of elastic band exercises designed to strengthen the rotator cuff muscles—all with limited success. His pain grew worse, and he had to stop pitching during practice entirely. One of the doctors referred him to an Applied Kinesiologist.

During the examination, Postural Analysis revealed that while standing relaxed, Frank's right hand turned more inwards than the left—so much so that the knuckles were actually facing forward. Gait Analysis demonstrated this same pattern. This led the Applied Kinesiologist to suspect that one of the external rotating muscles in the rotator cuff was not functioning properly. Muscle testing confirmed this suspicion. One of the muscles, the infraspinatus muscle, was physiologically inhibited. Also, several of Frank's ribs were found to be restricted when he moved his right arm upward. Rib restriction is a common factor in the pain and loss of mobility of the shoulder blade.

The scapulothoracic (ST) joint governs the shoulder blade. When it dysfunctions, the shoulder blade restricts causing the arm to move unnaturally to compensate and can cause damage to the other shoulder joints and the rotator cuff muscles. Also, the low or mid back muscles are affected as well. All of these factors contributed to Frank's condition of a rotator cuff dysfunction.

Treatment began with percussion therapy using a Vibracussor® to help relax the muscles of the mid back. This medical device uses a unique straight up and down movement with different frequencies to effectively release thickened areas of fascia (*myogelosis)* surrounding a muscle, bone or organ. Next, using a combination of chiropractic adjustments to restore normal movement to the affected ribs and an AK Scapula Mobilization Technique, the doctor managed to restore normal motion into the shoulder blade. Finally, the doctor used Origin/Insertion Technique to provide optimal facilitation of the affected rotator cuff muscle.

Frank noted immediate improvement in his arm and less pain when he engaged in the pitching motion that caused him to wince before the treatment. He required 8 treatments in total to restore normal function to his ribs and shoulder. He was given mid-back stretching exercises and told to continue with the elastic band exercises he was already doing, which would now work more effectively with the rotator cuff muscle facilitated. While he occasionally experienced some twinges when pitching, his condition was much improved. He continues to follow up for treatments during baseball's winter off-season.

Two Conditions Associated with a "Frozen Shoulder"

MARCUS, 60, was a high-powered and highly successful real estate developer in Manhattan. Over a period of three years, he had gradually lost mobility in both of his shoulders and arms. He knew something wasn't right, but he had no time to see a doctor. When his condition became so acute that he had to give up playing tennis, his one leisure activity, he made an appointment with an orthopedic doctor.

His orthopedic specialist diagnosed his problem as *adhesive capsulitis,* or "frozen shoulder." This condition is characterized by stiffness and pain in the shoulder that gradually progresses to the point where the arm can barely be moved, either actively by the patient or passively by anyone else, without pain. It is not uncommon for this condition to affect people with highly stressful lives. While no one knows the cause for this condition, it is usually linked to some event or series of events that impact the muscles and joints—slowly causing you to lose movement in your shoulder and arm if left untreated.

After nearly three years of standard treatments on his shoulders that included anti-inflammatories, chiropractic, medical massage, physical therapy, and cortisone shots—the pain had lessened, but the condition persisted. His orthopedic specialist suggested that he needed surgery. He refused to accept that diagnosis and sought out an alternative. His chiropractor referred him to an Applied Kinesiologist.

During the initial consultation, Marcus was clear that he wasn't interested in any kind of surgical intervention and wanted his condition cured. The doctor noted that Marcus was under a great deal of stress and assured him that he would not advise any invasive treatment; however, he could not guarantee that conservative treatments would be successful until he assessed Marcus' particular condition. Marcus reluctantly acknowledged this possibility, and the doctor began the examination.

Postural and Gait Analysis displayed that when Marcus stood, and especially when he walked, his body tightened up into a hunched position; similar to the stance of a wrestler about to attack his opponent. Given the amount of time that Marcus endured this condition and the failure of the medical treatments, the doctor surmised that there was an underlying cause of what his doctors had diagnosed as adhesive capsulitis.

During the examination, Marcus was unable to lift his arms enough for the doctor to do a full muscle testing protocol of the shoulder. The Applied Kinesiologist had to use his hands to feel for the shoulder adhesions and work them out manually with little to no effect. This clue sparked a thought in the Applied Kinesiologist's mind. Marcus's gait involved his constant tensing of the muscles of his ribcage. What if they had become so fatigued that they could not perform one of their chief functions: stabilizing the shoulder complex? The shoulder girdle sits on top of the ribs, and if the muscles of the ribcage are compromised, it will cause dysfunction in the shoulders.

Additional muscle testing of these muscles revealed that this was, in fact, the case. The source of the dysfunction was not in Marcus' shoulders but the muscles of his ribcage. The muscles were so weak from constant stress that they had all but collapsed. It didn't interfere with his breathing but affected his shoulders.

Knowing that the abdominals stabilize the ribcage and that any weakness or injury to these muscles can affect the ribs and, consequently, the shoulders, the doctor tested them as well. Marcus' abdominal muscles were also dysfunctional, in all likelihood, due to constant strain of stress-induced tension in the *wrestler position*. His love of playing tennis three times a week put additional strain on the abdominal muscles, as well as the other muscles of the ribcage, and most likely played a part in creating the "perfect storm" that led to his condition. This combined weakness of the abdominal and ribcage muscles was the actual source of Marcus' shoulder condition.

This was confirmed by the fact that when the doctor put his hands over the insertion of the abdominals on the ribcage and applied a slight downward pressure to support the action of the muscle, Marcus was able to raise his arms slightly higher than he could in years. Marcus was stunned.

The doctor shared his diagnosis: the dysfunction of the abdominals and the other rib muscles impacted his shoulder mobility and were the actual source of Marcus' problem. He said that the treatments would focus on restoring the proper function to them and, ultimately, resolve his condition.

The treatment involved the use of the Origin/Insertion Technique to facilitate the function of the muscles in the rib cage and abdominal region. Once facilitation was accomplished, the doctor would work on the shoulders.

After six sessions of working on Marcus' abdominals and his ribcage muscles, the doctor began to free up the two frozen shoulders. Proper abdominal exercises along with an exercise using a dumbbell known as a *pullover* were recommended to strengthen the ribcage muscles—once they were physiologically facilitated using AK procedures. After an additional three months of weekly treatments, Marcus had full motion restored, and he started physical therapy to strengthen his shoulder and abdominal muscles. The doctor recommended that he become more aware of his gait and posture, especially during stressful situations, and learn to take a deep breath and blow out forcibly instead of resuming his aggressive stance. Marcus regained his full mobility and resumed playing tennis.

* * *

DENNIS, 49, was a doctor of chiropractic with a very busy practice. He began to notice that his right arm was getting weaker but thought it was simply because he was fatigued from long hours and the many manipulations he did each day. However, he eventually lost the full function of his right arm. He could not raise his right arm more than horizontal to his body. Several doctors diagnosed him with adhesive capsulitis of his right shoulder and arm. He followed the full regimen of treatments including chiropractic, physical therapy, and acupuncture. However, his condition persisted; it was affecting his practice and his quality of life. He had heard about AK from several of his colleagues and decided to learn more about it by attending a seminar entitled, "Advanced Treatment for People with Shoulder Conditions." He was intrigued by the approach described in the seminar and decided to visit a local certified AK practitioner.

During the initial interview, Dennis described his condition. When asked if there was any trauma involving his shoulder, he related that he had been in a car accident a few years earlier where he felt like his ribcage and pelvis were "rattled" but hadn't experienced any pronounced aftereffects. However, when his practice had increased to the point that he spent prolonged hours sitting to do paperwork in addition to the usual amount during examination and treatment, his arm condition appeared and gradually grew worse.

Postural Analysis revealed a marked elevation of Dennis' right shoulder, and Gait Analysis revealed the same as well as little to no extension of the right arm behind him, which naturally should have occurred when he stepped forward with his right leg. He also had an unsteady stance when standing and walking.

Based on the information collected, the doctor surmised that the underlying cause of Dennis' condition was that the *latissimus muscle* (commonly called "the lat"), which governs the back and shoulder, had become physiologically inhibited. Muscle testing confirmed this inhibition *only* when Dennis was sitting. Since the lat originates in the pelvic region, this finding meant that the pelvis was unstable and was causing the physiological inhibition (weakness) of the lat and the resultant spasm, or *freezing up*, of his upper shoulder muscles.

In Dennis' case, his car accident could have contributed to the instability of his pelvis and did not present a problem until he began sitting for hours at a time. Because sitting puts additional pressure on the pelvis, this would explain the progression of Dennis' condition. This instability led to a reactive dysfunction of the lat muscle. Without the stabilizing factor of the lat, the upper shoulder muscles went into spasm which led to continuous pulling of the arm into the socket, thereby, "jamming it" and not allowing it to move in an upward direction.

While Dennis displayed symptoms of adhesive capsulitis, the source of his condition was not his shoulder but his unstable pelvis. The latissimus muscle tested physiologically inhibited only when he was sitting, but over time the residual spasms of the other shoulder muscles became constant and affected his shoulder and arm.

The doctor shared this diagnosis with Dennis. As a chiropractor, Dennis was able to fully appreciate this explanation. The treatments began with the doctor placing a sacroiliac belt over Dennis' pelvis for support. A sacroiliac belt is a thin supportive brace that goes directly over the pelvis above the groin. The application of the brace led to an immediate strengthening (physiological facilitation) of the latissimus and a corresponding relaxation of the spastic shoulder muscles and arm. Dennis was able to raise his arm fully over his head in less than 30 seconds of wearing the belt.

After three weeks of wearing the belt, especially when sitting for hours doing paperwork, and following several AK treatments consisting of a specific medical massage technique to restore normal function to the compromised muscles, Dennis went on to enjoy full use of his right arm.

* * *

These case studies illustrate the vital importance of treating the person experiencing a condition and not the condition itself. AK accomplishes this by its unique ability to discover the underlying weak (physiologically inhibited) muscle that is *causing* the tight (hypertonic) muscle(s) that most often receive the misguided focus as "being the problem" from patients and other practitioners.

Concerning Marcus and Dennis, they received the same diagnosis of *adhesive capsulitis* and yet, in each case, the standard treatment protocols were ineffective because the initial diagnosis was not the actual *source* of their individual conditions, and it overlooked the underlying muscular imbalances that were causing the debilitating restrictions. Regarding Letitia, her initial complaint was found to be linked to several sources. Applied Kinesiology resolves this common dilemma through the keen observation of movement coupled with specific muscle testing to treat each patient's individual condition successfully.

6

HIP AND KNEE CONDITIONS

According to the American Academy of Orthopedic Surgeons, there are currently over 600,000 knee replacement surgeries performed yearly in the US.[15] The Academy projects that by the year 2030 there will be over 3,000,000 Americans who will have full knee replacements yearly.[16] This study also projects that 500,000 Americans will need hip replacements as well.[16] Currently, over 7,000,000 Americans are living with an artificial hip or knee.[17]

Aside from the natural aging process and specific stresses placed on these joints in high impact activities such as sports, the two most probable causes of knee and hip conditions are linked to overweight and/or chronic misalignment. Our population suffers from pervasive obesity issues. Any additional pounds beyond your healthy weight wreak havoc on your knees and hips. For instance, just 10 extra pounds of body weight adds 40 pounds of pressure to your knees and other lower body joints—leading to serious conditions.

Most people do not have their knees and hips checked for proper alignment regularly or even when they experience pain. Conditions that could be cured with chiropractic and AK techniques are usually treated with anti-inflammatory drugs, both over-the-counter and prescription until the joints themselves deteriorate and require replacement. Owing to the failure to recognize the need for early intervention, it is not difficult to see why replacement surgery has become the treatment of last resort for so many people.

THE HIP

Along with the shoulder, the hip is one of only two ball and socket joints in the body and is considered the strongest. The hip joint consists of the pelvis and the thigh bone (femur). The femur is the longest and heaviest bone in the body and represents the pivoting point of your hip. The top end of the femur is rounded and fits into a socket-like structure in your pelvis. The hip socket, called the acetabulum, is lined with a smooth, rubbery material known as cartilage. Healthy cartilage provides for frictionless motion and keeps the lubricating synovial fluid safely in the hip as well as most of your other joints.

For the hip joint to accomplish all the varied movements and provide the necessary strength to maintain healthy bodily structure, your hip has approximately 20 muscles to ensure a wide range of motion and to provide for the necessary stability. One set of these muscles lifts one leg while another set stabilizes the other leg that is in the stationary position. Because of the interrelationship of these muscle groups, any imbalance can lead to hip problems.

The most commonly known condition relating to the femur/pelvic bone is known as a "broken hip." It arises from fractures to the femur and/or pelvic bone. Any traumatic impact to the hip can cause a fracture at any age. Falls are the most prevalent cause of a broken hip, especially in older individuals. Over 300,000 people age 65 and older are hospitalized for hip fractures each year due to falls.[18]

Another contributing factor to the high percentage of hip injuries in this age group is the increasing brittleness of bones as we age. Diminished amounts of calcium and other minerals in older people can cause these bones to weaken, leaving them prone to fracture. Attention to nutrition throughout our lives is vital to keeping our bones strong. Taking bone-strengthening nutrients, such as calcium, magnesium, boron, copper, vitamin K2 and vitamin D3, will prevent many serious hip-related problems. You can also help your joints by taking a daily dose of lubricating and cartilage supporting nutrients such as hyaluronic acid, glucosamine sulfate, gelatin, and omega 3 oils. You also want to keep your bones strong by doing weight-bearing exercises such as strength training, balance exercises, and walking, along with muscle stretching to achieve a full range of motion.

However, while a broken hip is the most serious condition, there are other chronic conditions such as bursitis and arthritis that cause discomfort and deterioration. The most common factor that can cause these conditions is an imbalance of the muscles surrounding the joint—resulting in misalignment of the bones themselves. Once the bones are out of alignment, they can wear away at the cartilage. As this natural lubricating tissue diminishes, the bones rub against each other causing more inflammation in the joint.

Bursitis represents irritation of the bursa, the sac-like cushion filled with synovial fluid located between bone and soft tissues such as muscles, tendons, and skin. When irritated, they become inflamed and cause pain. There are over 150 bursae distributed throughout your body and are found in nearly every joint. Swelling of the bursa, as well as the surrounding muscles (myositis) and tendons (tendonitis), is usually an acute reaction to a misalignment of the bones comprising the joint and not simply the result of aging or overuse.

Arthritis literally means inflammation of the joint(s). This painful condition is usually the result of a chronic misalignment of the bones. If left untreated, this misalignment leads to the loss of cartilage. Severe conditions such as osteoarthritis, if not treated early, can cause chronic pain and problems with mobility.

Another syndrome associated with hip problems (and joint problems in general) is a phenomenon known as "immobilization degeneration," whereby a joint will break down if it is not moved through its full range of motion regularly. This occurs because cartilage needs joint motion to stay healthy. Any joint not moved will begin to experience *chondrocyte* loss within one day. Chondrocytes are the cells that repair and regenerate the cartilage in a joint. Numerous studies have shown that this condition is becoming more prevalent in our increasingly sedentary society. Very few people move the hip joint any further than is necessary to go from sitting to standing positions. The full range of motion needs to involve forward and backward movement, internal/external rotation, and side-to-side movements—preferably while standing. Daily attention to this full range of motion with proper exercise will help prevent hip problems resulting from immobilization degeneration.

Applied Kinesiology supports a full complement of preventative efforts to avoid hip problems. As mentioned above, keeping the hip complex limber and strong, by doing weight-bearing exercises such as deep squats, lunges, and walking; in addition to balancing exercises and muscle stretching, will maintain a full range of motion and balance. Regular visits to your AK professional will ensure that your hips are in their proper alignment. But the most important thing to remember is to be in touch with your body. As with most health conditions, the body will signal to you if there is a problem through one of its most effective and natural alert systems—pain.

Paying attention to pain is particularly important to hip and general joint health. Discomfort usually indicates that our body is not functioning properly. If we ignore this early warning sign, conditions left untreated can wear away existing cartilage and tissues, leaving no other option but surgery. While synthetic drugs help us cope with pain, they often can give us a false sense of well-being. When you are medicated, you become numb to this important indicator and can put off addressing the underlying issue. Without proper intervention as early as possible, simple problems can become major ones. Applied Kinesiology does not rely on numbing agents. It focuses on the treatment of the source of the pain to help the body heal itself by restoring proper function.

Conditions Associated with Hip Problems

ROSA, 32, was a mother of two young children aged 9 and 5. Her days were busy running the household, chasing her children around, and doing a great deal of bending, lifting and stooping over. Soon after a family vacation to Disney World, she experienced a throbbing, sharp pain in her right hip. She tried ice, heat, yoga, and over-the-counter medications. Nothing helped. The pain became so severe that she went to a local walk-in clinic. The clinic staff suggested getting a series of X-rays and MRIs to check if there were any fractures or hip disease that might be causing the pain. The results were negative for any kind of break or other pathology. Not a fan of traditional medicine, she avoided seeing an orthopedic specialist and found her way to a doctor of chiropractic who was also certified in AK.

During her consultation, Rosa related to the AK doctor that the hip pain started after the family trip to Disney World. The doctor asked if she went on any particularly bumpy rides. She had not. Further inquiry led to the discovery that her five-year-old son liked to be picked up and carried a great deal of the time. Her son weighed 40 lbs., a significant amount of weight to be bending over and twisting to lift regardless of much she loved holding him. Typically, she would also push her hip out to the side to support her son, taking some of the weight off of her arms and shoulders, as she carried him. This position is common for parents, mothers in particular.

Gait Analysis revealed that her right hip was noticeably elevated when she walked. It was also higher than the right when she stood still in Postural Analysis. This generally indicates a weakness of the gluteus medius muscle, which connects the pelvis to the femur. As we said earlier, the muscles surrounding the hip must perform different functions to either move or stabilize the bones and joints. For example, if you are taking a step with your right leg, your right gluteus medius muscle brings your walking leg outwards, while the opposite gluteus medius on the left stabilizes the hip on the side of the leg that is on the ground.

In Rosa's case, this muscle appeared to be compromised. Muscle testing confirmed this inhibition of the gluteus medius and was linked to a slight misalignment of her fifth lumbar vertebra just above the pelvis. When out of alignment, the vertebra puts pressure on the superior gluteal nerve which controls the gluteus medius and causes it to become physiologically inhibited. This muscular inhibition allowed her hipbone to rotate outwards and forward, causing the sharp hip pain Rosa experienced. The doctor concluded that this was the source of Rosa's pain.

The Applied Kinesiologist performed a precise chiropractic adjustment to realign the fifth lumbar bone to allow the nerve to function properly. Then he made two joint realignment manipulations on her hip to restore its proper movement. When Rosa got off of the treatment table, she noticed relief from the sharp, piercing pain.

The doctor gave Rosa hip exercises and stretches to do at home including rolling her hips inwards and outwards for a minute before exiting the bed in the morning to warm up the joints before starting her day of bending, squatting, stooping, and lifting. He also advised her to avoid lifting her son, unless absolutely necessary, until she was completely healed. After six treatments to ensure that the bones in the lower back and pelvis maintained their proper positions and that her gluteus medius muscle was working well—she was free of pain and able to resume all the various physical activities of her day—including picking up her son.

* * *

ERIC, 50, was a Grammy Award-winning music producer. Always an active person, his increasing success compounded his workload to where he frequently sat for long periods at his desk, sometimes up to twelve hours at a stretch. He no longer exercised and was beginning to put on some weight. He began to experience a dull ache in his left hip that progressed to a sharp pain down his leg. The pain became so bad that he had to walk with a cane. Eric went to his regular doctor, who sent him to have X-rays and MRIs taken. The results were inconclusive, so the doctor prescribed the over-the-counter pain suppressant ibuprofen and advised Eric to begin getting up from his chair and moving more often. However, the pain continued. Eric saw an orthopedic specialist, who diagnosed his condition as osteoarthritis based on his symptoms, X-rays, and MRIs. He recommended arthroscopic hip surgery.

One of the most common ways traditional medicine addresses joint problems is arthroscopic surgery—a minimally invasive procedure wherein a slight incision is made to the affected area. An arthroscope is inserted which allows the surgeon to view the internal condition and perform surgery with increased precision.

However, Eric was resistant to having surgery because his father had died from complications related to hip surgery. He sought an alternative and visited a highly recommended medical general practitioner who was licensed in chiropractic and certified in AK.

After an in-depth interview, the physician inspected the medical records and agreed that Eric's symptoms indicated that the orthopedist's diagnosis seemed correct. However, the fundamental cause of the osteoarthritis remained unclear. The doctor believed that once the origin of the problem was found, Eric could make a more informed decision on how to proceed.

The doctor's exam began with Postural Analysis which was unremarkable, and Gait Analysis which revealed that when Eric walked, his left foot pointed dramatically out to the side. This excessive rotation appeared to be coming from his hip—indicating a possible spasm or fascial shortening associated with a dysfunction of the piriformis muscle. This muscle is located in the buttock and serves to help turn the thigh bone outwards.

The doctor applied the AK procedure of Stretch Inhibition Technique to uncover the all-too-common phenomenon whereby the fascial covering of a muscle has become so tight that it inhibits healthy muscle function. As the doctor suspected, the piriformis was indeed physiologically inhibited. This discovery led to the diagnosis that the underlying cause of Eric's condition was piriformis syndrome.

Piriformis syndrome is common in people who sit for long periods. Prolonged sitting is a highly stressful position for the hip and can cause a slight separation of the pelvis. When this happens, the piriformis muscle goes into spasm trying to hold the joint together. This spasm and resultant fascial shortening of the piriformis muscle can compress the sciatic nerve—the largest nerve in the body that runs beneath it—resulting in piercing, paralyzing pain down the leg. Unfortunately, this slight separation in the pelvis does not show up on X-rays or MRIs. Due to the inflammation and painful symptoms it causes, it is often simply diagnosed as osteoarthritis.

Using TL, the doctor recognized that Eric's hipbone was slightly out of alignment as well. He utilized the AK diagnostic technique of Joint Challenging, wherein the doctor gently pushes the bone in question in different directions to see which direction causes an impact to the patient's nervous system—temporarily inhibiting any tested muscle. After the direction of misalignment was determined, the examination continued by testing the various hip related muscles to ascertain which muscles were weak enough to cause the misalignment. Once the AK practitioner discovered the inhibited muscles, the realignment process could begin. The doctor started with a deep medical massage using a Vibracussor® to lengthen the fascia and restore the tightened muscle to full function; then a specific chiropractic adjustive technique known as Joint Traction, in which the femur is rotated in and gently coaxed back into place, was performed. Once properly aligned and supported by a strong piriformis muscle, Eric's pain was greatly reduced.

To maintain the alignment, the doctor recommended a sacroiliac belt to stabilize the region as well as a regimen of getting up for ten minutes every hour. Also, Eric was to take daily 20-minute walking breaks at least twice a day and perform stretching exercises. The Applied Kinesiologist also recommended natural anti-inflammatory nutrients, specifically omega 3 oils and the herbs ginger and boswellia, to help with the hip and sciatic pain. Additionally, he was advised to take a nutritional supplement containing hyaluronic acid and glucosamine sulfate to aid the joint in its healing and lower the possibility of this condition recurring in the future.

Eric had eight more sessions to fully resolve the pain. He was instructed to continue to wear the belt during waking hours, particularly when he was sitting for prolonged periods. The changes in lifestyle helped him lose weight, which contributed to his total recovery. Eric remains pain-free without any surgical intervention. He often substitutes playing a game of basketball with his wife for one of his daily walks. Eric keeps his cane in the corner of his recording studio as a reminder to get up for ten minutes every hour.

* * *

SAL, 71, was the owner of a large chain of pizzerias. He worked long hours, predominately standing most of the time. He had always enjoyed good health, but over a period of about two years, he started to suffer from sharp pain in his right hip and buttocks. The constant pain would become nearly bearable if he took frequent breaks—something he had not needed to do for his entire life. After a few minutes, the pain would subside, and Sal would resume working again. Eventually, he found it difficult to maintain his grueling schedule and had to take increasingly frequent breaks.

Not one to visit doctors, Sal researched his symptoms online and came to the conclusion that he was suffering from *sciatica*, a condition in which severe pain affects the back, hip, buttocks and outer side of the leg from compression of the sciatic nerve. He began self-medicating with the over-the-counter pain suppressant ibuprofen. While it helped to make the pain manageable, the condition continued to worsen. As with many people who had enjoyed good health all their lives, he thought he could "tough it out" without wasting time in some doctor's office.

Sal's son was concerned about his father as he watched him work while in pain. Knowing that Sal would not agree to visit a specialist, he suggested that his father visit his general practitioner who was certified in AK. He guaranteed his dad that there would be no talk of anything that would keep him from the business, such as surgery. Sal knew that this doctor had helped his son with some back problems and agreed to "talk" to him.

In the patient interview, the doctor uncovered several critical factors regarding Sal's lifestyle that helped shed light on his condition. Sal was proud of the fact that he maintained the same punishing schedule that he had as a young man. As a hands-on owner, he never sat still. For example, he would be in the office with the accountants and managers; then go to his office and be on the phone with vendors; then he would go the loading area and help with loading or unloading trucks. He even pitched in helping to make pizzas.

Sal mentioned that walking aggravated his condition so much that he even had to cut short his walks with his dog, which were apparently his greatest source of pleasure outside of work. He even went so far as to stop his water consumption, which was limited to begin with, to minimize having to walk down the hall to use the restroom.

As his pain increased, he mentioned that he had changed his approximately 25-year-old bed mattress to a soft, foam one thinking it would help him to rest easier. Unfortunately, it did not; soft mattresses often contribute to and can even adversely affect healthy muscle and spine function.

These might sound like routine aspects of any busy person's life, but in Sal's case, they were crucial to diagnosing his condition.

Gait and Postural Analysis revealed a slight lowering of his right ribcage, which in itself did not seem to explain his sharp hip pain. The doctor referred Sal for X-rays of his lower back, pelvis, and hip and told him to return in a week with the films and the report.

The following week, Sal returned begrudgingly with X-rays in hand. The radiologist report mentioned that the lumbar spine, pelvis and hip were all within normal limits of alignment and that there were no fractures or pathologies. Sal emphatically asked, "So, if everything is okay, why am I in so much damn pain?"

"Actually Sal," replied his doctor, "this report just means that there is nothing wrong with your bones or spine. Let's discuss it further."

The doctor questioned Sal more deeply about how the pain manifested daily. "The pain gets really bad after I walk about two blocks with my dog in the morning," he said. "Then it goes on all day at work." The proverbial light bulb went off in the doctor's mind that he was not having Sal walk long enough when he was performing Gait Analysis for him to experience the pain. The doctor replied, "Sal grab your coat. We are going outside."

Sal started walking up and down the street in front of the office with his doctor close behind him. At one block, the doctor noted that Sal started to lean noticeably to his left as if he was carrying a heavy load with his left hand. Incredibly, exactly at the two-block mark, he started limping.

Back in the office, the doctor put Sal face down on the treatment table, and to pinpoint the cause of what he observed, the AK practitioner palpated the right quadratus lumborum muscle. The quadratus lumborum muscle sits in the flank area over the kidney and connects the ribs to the pelvis. It is the deepest of the abdominal muscles, serves to stabilize the pelvis and spine area as well as the 12th rib, and is important for bending to each side. The doctor felt a small nodule which could cause dysfunction of the muscle.

He then had Sal lie face up, tested the muscle, and found it apparently normal. However, having felt what appeared to be a trigger point, he sensed that something could be affecting normal muscle function. Using the Stretch Inhibition Technique, the doctor stretched the muscle and immediately tested it again. It became grossly inhibited. Weakness in this muscle indicated that the fascia surrounding it had tightened and created a trigger point over time. After walking more than a block or approximately 600 feet, this fascial shortening became aggravated, and it caused Sal to have severe pain and weakness in the hip and leg.

"So, it's not sciatica," Sal said.

"No. Your symptoms are similar, but it has nothing to do with your sciatic nerve. It has to do with your lower back muscle."

"So, where do we go from here?"

The doctor assured him the treatments would be limited, non-invasive, would not impact Sal's schedule, and could start right now. Sal agreed.

First, the doctor applied pressure and focused vibration for one minute on the trigger point, using a hand-held device known as a "Nimmo® T." This device is shaped like the letter T with the horizontal part being held in the doctor's hand and the vertical part, which has a cushion on the end, being placed onto the trigger point. The pressure and vibration help to break the trigger point up and allow the muscle to heal. Sal felt pain initially, but as the trigger point disappeared, so did the pain.

Then treatment continued with the placing of an ice pack on the quadratus muscle and then slowly stretching and lengthening the muscle/fascia complex as the doctor pulled the patient's two legs to the left side, going a little farther each time. This technique is known as Cool and Stretch and relieves the fascial shortening. By applying this technique, the doctor was able to restore the muscle to its proper function and prevent the pain from recurring. When Sal left the office, his pain and weakness had greatly diminished.

Sal required four additional treatments for this condition. He was instructed to replace his soft foam mattress with a firmer one to stabilize his spine and relax his muscles while he slept. The doctor taught him stretches for his quadratus lumborum muscle and instructed him to drink more water to help keep the muscle supple. After a few weeks, Sal was no longer in pain, and he could continue to run his business at his usual hectic pace and resume his long walks with his dog without any problem.

The Knee

The knee is generally considered to be the largest joint in your body. It is comprised of four bones: the tibia or shin bone; the femur or thigh bone; patella or knee cap and, to a lesser degree, the fibula or calf bone. The knee must endure the force of 1.5 times your body weight when you walk on flat ground. The pressure on each knee increases to double or triple your body weight when you go up or down stairs and four to five times your weight when you squat down. For example, if you weigh 200 lbs., your knee is exposed to 350 lbs. with every step you take on flat ground, up to 600 lbs. going upstairs, and up to 1,000 lbs. each time you squat down to pick something up off the floor. It is no wonder that this kind of daily stress, unless properly distributed, can lead to knee problems over time.

As does your hip and other joints, your knee functions normally thanks to the protein-rich synovial fluid which lubricates the bones and helps prevent wear and tear. It is important to eat high-quality protein to maintain the needed levels of synovial fluid. Your body requires protein to function. Unless your diet supplies high-quality protein, your system will take it from other tissues in your body, including the synovial fluid, which could affect its ability to lubricate the joints fully.

The knee is one of several hinge joints in your body that include the elbow and ankle. However, it has one unique quality—it not only bends, but it also slightly rotates. This additional rotary movement is critical to the knee's full range of motion, which enables us to maintain our mobility in such varied functions as standing, walking, running, squatting, climbing, kicking, and dancing.

Like most joints, the knee has ligaments inside the synovial joint capsule that regulate knee function and joint alignment. One set includes the anterior cruciate ligament (ACL) and posterior cruciate ligament (PCL). These keep the bone at the bottom part of the joint (the tibia) from slipping forward or backward. There are strong ligaments on each side of the knee known as collateral ligaments that are responsible for restricting side-to-side movement. The knee also has articular cartilage covering the ends of the bones and figure eight-shaped shock absorbers known as the meniscus to cushion the joint, especially during high-impact activities such as running and jumping.

Despite the roles of the previously mentioned ligaments and approximately 12 muscles that keep the knee bones in place, the fact that the two largest bones—the femur and the tibia—are basically stacked on top of each other to form the majority of the joint, misalignments often occur and are a common cause of most knee problems. If left untreated, these misalignments can eventually lead to painful conditions such as arthritis, sudden knee weakness known as "trick knee syndrome," injury to the meniscus or the ACL, and degeneration of cartilage. The most common symptoms include sharp knee pain, stiffness, difficulty in walking, climbing stairs, standing for long periods, kneeling, and squatting.

As stated above, the portion of the knee joint that is most susceptible to this misalignment is where the large femur and tibia bones meet. If the muscles are strong, they help to prevent misalignment. However, if the muscles are not functioning optimally, the ligaments can become compromised or torn, and the resulting slippage out of position can sometimes cause irreversible damage unless diagnosed early.

Similar to certain hip conditions, this misalignment in the knee can be so subtle that it does not show up on X-rays or MRIs. Often it is not until the pain gets so acute that people feel the need to seek professional help. Initially, medical doctors and orthopedic specialists will treat the symptoms with pain-suppressing or anti-inflammatory drugs. Unfortunately, by that time, substantial damage may have already progressed to the point that surgery becomes the only option.

AK takes another approach. Through functional muscle testing techniques, the dysfunction of the muscle groups and bony misalignments can be detected early. Once these muscles are strengthened and the bones aligned properly, any pain or subsequent long-term damage can be prevented.

Conditions Associated with Sharp Knee Pain

PAUL, 28, was a Secret Service agent suffering from symptoms related to what he thought was a sprain of his right knee. For several months, he endured the pain and often experienced sudden weakness in his knee that caused him to stumble briefly. He decided to make an appointment with an orthopedist who specialized in knee problems.

After examining him, the doctor sent Paul for X-rays and an MRI. The reports stated that there was a slight tear of the medial meniscus. The doctor said that it could take several weeks of complete bed rest to see if it healed on its own; or Paul could have arthroscopic surgery, which would require a sustained recovery period and PT. Paul couldn't afford to take the time off necessary for either of these treatment options. His partner suggested that he get another opinion from an entirely different perspective and suggested that he see an Applied Kinesiologist whom he knew. Skeptical, but seeing no harm in a second opinion, Paul agreed.

When Paul entered the office, the doctor could readily see that the patient was favoring the injured knee. During the consult, Paul mentioned that he was wearing a light knee brace under his slacks which seemed to strengthen the knee. The doctor asked him to remove the brace and walk down the hall. Gait analysis revealed that Paul could not fully straighten his right leg and compensated by slightly swinging his hip to move forward.

"Do you have any pain in your hip?" the doctor asked.

Paul was surprised at the question. "How did you know my hip has been starting to ache?"

"I could see by the way you were compensating for your knee with your hip when you walk. This additional pressure causes some pain there. The knee and hip represent two moveable ends of the same bone. A problem in one will eventually lead to a problem in the other one."

Paul nodded, acknowledging the common sense of the statement, while the doctor proceeded to read the X-ray and MRI reports. The reports showed some inflammation and a slight meniscus tear.

The examination revealed that Paul could not fully bend or straighten his knee without sharp pain. Muscle testing showed a marked inhibition of two key knee muscles: the vastus medialis (inner knee), which is part of the quadriceps, and the sartorius muscle. AK Joint Challenging uncovered that the tibia was misaligned as well, rotating outwards and to the side. These factors appeared to be the main cause of the problem, including the meniscus tear.

The Applied Kinesiologist shared his diagnosis with his patient. "Will I still need surgery?" Paul asked.

"No. I don't think surgery is the answer to this problem in your case. We can do the treatment right in this office, but it might take several visits to treat it. We can begin right now if you like."

Paul agreed, and the doctor got to work. He began with the AK technique of Origin/Insertion to facilitate and restore normal function to the injured portion of the quadriceps and sartorius muscles. Then, using two specific chiropractic adjustments to the tibia bone, he restored the knee to its proper alignment. Using his thumb, the doctor adjusted the medial meniscus to re-establish an optimal relationship of the meniscus to the now properly aligned knee joint. Paul felt some relief after this first treatment.

The doctor gave Paul exercises to strengthen the medial quadriceps and sartorius muscles and instructed him to keep wearing the knee brace until he was completely free of pain. The doctor also recommended a nutritional supplement containing hyaluronic acid, glucosamine sulfate, and chondroitin sulfate to help the joint to heal and gelatin capsules for additional help with any damage to the meniscus.

After ten short visits over two months, his knee pain had completely dissipated. Paul keeps up the exercises and the supplements to prevent any further problems, and he remains fully functional.

* * *

ANTHONY, 17, was the star running back on his high school football team. He was in his senior year, and his team was having a great season. His coach was confident that he could get a football scholarship to college. However, by the middle of the season, Anthony had developed severe right knee pain and had to stop playing. Concerned about his health and his college future, Anthony's parents took him to an orthopedist who had an MRI done. The results were inconclusive, but the doctor felt that the likely reason for his pain was damage to the anterior cruciate ligament (ACL)—a condition that would require surgery. Anthony and his family were devastated. His recovery from the surgery would take him out of the remaining games for the entire season. It could mean the end of his hopes for a scholarship, as the college scouts were beginning to visit high school prospects.

Upon hearing the diagnosis, Anthony's coach was concerned. He knew how important the season was to Anthony and his family. He suggested that perhaps the condition was not as serious as the doctor said and could be treated without surgery. He shared his own story about a severe lower back problem he had suffered several years back. All the specialists said he needed surgery. It would have required him to take a leave of absence, so he explored his other options. He got in touch with an Applied Kinesiologist who specialized in sports injuries. The doctor had cured him without surgery. He recommended that Anthony see this doctor for a second opinion. Anthony and his parents agreed to give it try.

During the interview, the doctor asked if Anthony had experienced any trauma to his knee—he had not. Then Anthony related that, at first, the pain came on gradually when he began a run during practice but then became so intense that he had to stop running. However, he didn't have the pain while walking or standing. The doctor looked at the MRI report and noted that the radiologist stated that the image was so blurred by the level of inflammation in the area that it was not possible to see a full tear in the ligament. The AK specialist knew that if there were a serious ACL tear, Anthony would have experienced pain when walking as well as running. This observation plus the fact that most ACL tears have a history of trauma or a sudden incidence of sharp pain or "popping" led the doctor to suspect that there could be something else causing the condition.

Postural Analysis revealed Anthony to be slightly "flat-footed" (also known as ankle pronation or pes planus) on the right. Gait Analysis confirmed that Anthony was able to walk without pain. He had Anthony run down the hall, and, almost immediately, he felt the sharp pain in the front of his knee. The examination advanced to the muscle-testing portion, and the doctor could not find any muscle inhibition or joint misalignment of the knee joint itself. Upon further testing, the doctor uncovered a physiological inhibition of the tibialis posterior muscle along with a *stretch inhibition* of the tibialis anterior muscle which is in the front of the tibia. This problem is a common cause of the condition runners suffer from known as *shin splints.*

When asked about this, Anthony related that he did have a case of shin splints before the season began. He had eased up on some of his conditioning training, and the pain stopped. But as the season progressed, the knee pain began and slowly worsened. The doctor surmised that this information pointed to a possible problem in the relationship between the tibia (shin bone) and the talus (ankle bone). The tibia extends down the leg to connect to the talus bone which, in effect, represents the foundation of the knee joint. Additional muscle testing of the muscles surrounding the talus bone indicated that they were so severely restricted that Anthony could not physically pull his foot upward without feeling the sharp pain in his knee. This movement is known as dorsiflexion and occurs with greater repetition and intensity with running than with walking.

The doctor explained that since the ankle and knee are connected to the tibia, any dysfunction in the ankle could affect the biomechanics of the knee. In Anthony's case, the inhibition (weakness) of the tibialis posterior muscle—which lies under the calf and whose function is to hold the "ankle mortise" joint in place—combined with a fascial shortening of both the tibialis anterior and calf muscles caused Anthony's ankle to become locked in a position that shifted his weight forward. When he ran, Anthony's ankle bone (talus) needed to glide backward and not remain forward as it did.

This *ankle* impingement resulted in inflammation and the pain in his *knee*. It was the shin and calf muscles in the ankle that needed to be treated to relieve the problem. No surgery was required.

Needless to say, Anthony and his parents were relieved to receive this diagnosis and, yet, were a bit skeptical. How could the orthopedic specialist diagnose a condition that required surgery when it was not required? The AK specialist explained that since the vast majority of knee problems in athletes result from tears in the ACL, and the MRI had shown so much inflammation in the area, it was logical for the doctor to assume that this was the problem. Anthony and his parents were satisfied with the doctor's explanation and agreed to start with the treatment right away.

Applying the AK Origin/Insertion Technique, the doctor restored proper function to the inhibited tibialis posterior muscle in the back of the leg and ankle. He relieved the tightening of fascia surrounding the tibialis anterior muscle on the front of the shin and to the calf muscles with specific muscle manipulation. Then, he employed chiropractic adjustments to several lumbar vertebrae in the lower back through which the nerves that control these muscles travel. Increased pressure on these vertebrae, in all likelihood, arose due to compensating for the talus condition and was affecting the nerves, contributing to muscle inhibition and subsequent pain.

The doctor then asked Anthony to lie face down on the examination table. He adjusted the ankle bone to restore normal motion to the joint. When the doctor delivered the chiropractic adjustment to the ankle bone, there was a loud "click," indicating that the built-up pressure had been released. Anthony felt immediate relief from the constant tightness in his ankle that usually accompanied his knee pain when he ran.

The doctor instructed Anthony to get up and walk down the hall. Just as before, he stated he felt fine. Instead of having the patient run down the hall again, the doctor this time accompanied Anthony outside and instructed the patent to run down the block. Anthony tentatively began with a jog, then sprinted down the street and returned, exclaiming, "The pain is gone!"

Anthony required only this one office treatment and a follow-up visit a few weeks later. The doctor taught Anthony exercises to strengthen the tibialis anterior muscles in the front of his shins and to follow them with calf stretches for 30-60 seconds for each leg to help prevent impingement of the ankle joint in the future.

The follow-up examination revealed that the ankle joint remained in place, and the knee pain had completely disappeared. Fully recovered, Anthony played the remainder of the season and was awarded the scholarship.

* * *

MARIA, 36, led a busy life as a mother, wife and the director of a philanthropic foundation. Basically, she rarely sat down, except at family meals or to drive. She exercised regularly at her gym and ate a healthy diet. Her daughter had joined the school soccer team, and Maria had begun practicing soccer kicks with her most afternoons. Then one day she felt a sharp pain deep in her left knee after getting up from a chair after dinner. She took a few ibuprofen pills, but the pain continued. She stopped exercising at the gym and practicing kicks with her daughter, hoping that the pain would disappear. However, the pain persisted for weeks. It was particularly acute when she climbed stairs.

She went to see her general practitioner, who had X-rays taken. The films did not reveal any fractures or other pathology in her knee or leg. He recommended that she see an orthopedist. The specialist looked at the X-rays and examined her but again could not find any indication of ligament damage, one of the most common causes of knee pain. Since there were no clinical signs of ligament or meniscal damage on the numerous orthopedic tests that he performed, he did not feel that MRIs were warranted. Having no clear-cut diagnosis, the doctor suggested that she try PT. Maria went to PT three times a week for a month. Her pain did not diminish. A friend of hers recommended that she see the AK doctor that she was seeing, who was helping her with a shoulder problem, for another opinion before going back to the orthopedist.

During her initial visit with the AK practitioner, Maria described her condition and the ways she was told to address it. Nothing was helping her. The doctor asked if she had any recent physical trauma. She said she hadn't, but after a brief pause, she then shared the fact that she had suffered a severe gymnastic injury when she was 13. In gym class, she had done a handstand and went into a split. However, she had landed incorrectly, her left leg hit the mat hard, and she felt severe pain in her left knee. She was rushed to the hospital, where they discovered that she had dislocated her kneecap (patella). The doctors put it back into place and placed her leg in a hard cast for six weeks. She was instructed to have PT after the cast was removed but never went. Over the years, Maria noticed that her left knee always seemed weaker than her right, and her left front thigh muscle was smaller than her right—no matter how much she exercised to build it up. However, she never experienced any knee pain.

After looking at the radiology and orthopedic reports, and hearing Maria relate no recent incident of trauma and no "locking or snapping" of the knee, the doctor agreed that there didn't appear to be any reason to suspect pathology, meniscal damage or ligament tears. With the patient sitting during the consultation as well as when standing (Postural Analysis), the doctor noted that Maria rotated her left foot slightly outwards. During Gait Analysis, the Applied Kinesiologist immediately noticed how much more dramatically her left foot turned out in stark contrast to her right, which pointed perfectly straight. Because this turning out of the foot can be associated with the knee (a rotated tibia), the doctor surmised that there must be some issue with her popliteus muscle. This muscle is located in the back of the knee under the gastrocnemius, one of the calf muscles. The role of the popliteus muscle is to aid in the flexing of the knee and in keeping the foot in a proper forward position. The popliteus muscle is critical in flexing the knee when you first bend your leg to move from a standing to a sitting or squatting position and when you begin walking or running.

Sure enough, when the doctor tested Maria's left popliteus muscle, he discovered that it was inhibited. Additional functional muscle testing revealed that Maria's left quadriceps muscle was also inhibited and probably had been since her injury in her teens. Her doctor explained that, when a muscle is injured and left untreated, it remains *physiologically inhibited* and won't respond to exercise. This is why her left thigh muscle remained smaller than the right, despite her strengthening exercises at the gym.

Further examination revealed that Maria's tibia bone, the large bone at the bottom of the knee, had rotated outwards slightly. Her doctor explained that this is a common condition that appears to be caused by people habitually turning their foot out when getting out of a chair or car. Since Maria's quadriceps muscle had remained compromised for decades after her gymnastic accident, she probably developed this same habit.

The doctor asked Maria to describe the gym routine that she had followed before she had the recent knee problem and found nothing problematic about her workouts. Then she shared that she started practicing soccer kicks with her daughter. The doctor asked her to demonstrate how she kicked the soccer ball, as well as how she got up from a chair. In both instances, her doctor observed that she turned her leg out from the knee joint instead of turning the entire thigh out from the hip.

"I don't understand why I'm getting the pain now after all these years if I do this all the time," Maria asked.

"People generally do not realize that it is not the 100th straw that breaks the proverbial camel's back, it is the preceding 99. This could have happened at any time," the doctor responded. "In your case, the added stress from turning your foot out to kick the soccer ball with the inside of the foot was the final straw that exacerbated the situation, resulting in the knee pain."

"But I practiced with my daughter for weeks before the pain started."

"Yes. However, when you twisted your foot outwards one night to push up from the dinner table, the tibia bone must have rotated too far due to the inability of the muscle to maintain it in proper alignment, and the pain began. Once we strengthen the muscle and restore proper alignment, the pain should subside."

Treatment to restore normal function included the use of Origin/Insertion Technique to the inhibited quadriceps and popliteus muscles. The doctor performed a precise chiropractic adjustment consisting of a gentle counter-rotation manipulation to return the rotated tibia bone to its proper position, effectively aligning the knee joint. After the first treatment, Maria got up from a chair and was able to do a deep full squat for the first time in weeks—without pain.

The Applied Kinesiologist gave her the specific exercise of twisting her whole body while standing on one leg to strengthen the popliteus muscle at least once a day. He suggested that she take start taking natural anti-inflammatory supplements, such as boswellia, rutin, and ginger—and to apply arnica gel to the knee to limit any swelling caused by the shifting of her knee bone.

To avoid a recurrence of her condition, the AK practitioner instructed Maria to change the way she got up from a chair or car seat by using her entire lower body to turn her leg out from the hip and pelvis, and not from the knee or foot. Also, he suggested that she visualize kicking the soccer ball by twisting her entire lower body, not only her leg. When the pain subsided, she could practice her kicks. She agreed to follow this regimen.

Maria required a total of eight treatments to restore her alignment and muscle strength permanently. She continues to pursue her busy life and practice soccer pain-free.

* * *

The hip and knee are the two largest joints in your body and are nearly constantly in use. Due to the amount of stress they experience, they are particularly susceptible to misalignment of the bones and to ligament injuries, both of which can lead to acute pain and chronic degenerative problems when left untreated. The increased frequency of hip and knee surgery, including replacements, stems from the failure of people to seek help as soon as they feel recurring pain or stiffness in these major joints. Attention to the body's early warning signals, such as pain or mobility issues, can make all the difference to your joint health.

Recently, the Stanford University School of Medicine conducted a symposium stressing the vital importance of the 25 "high yield bedside maneuvers" with particular attention to hip and knee exams.[19] This symposium underscored the fact that specialists have become overly dependent on radiological diagnostic tests, which do not always allow for precise diagnoses. They need to be supported by traditional assessment tools, such as hands-on examination and talking to the patient.

As we've seen in the case studies in this chapter, high-tech diagnostic tests such as X-rays and MRIs often miss the underlying cause of hip and knee problems. The precise diagnostic approach of AK through physical examination and muscle testing techniques can be an integral component in uncovering the root cause of hip and knee pain. After proper diagnosis of the underlying joint dysfunction, AK's unique methods to restore the body's natural function, particularly in these complex joint issues, can prevent unnecessary surgical procedures or reliance on painkillers and help you to enjoy a lifetime of pain-free mobility.

7

ANKLE AND FOOT CONDITIONS

The ankle and foot complete the body's mobility system. They serve to support us in standing, walking, running, climbing and just about every move we make. Along with the knee, these complex joints help us absorb and distribute the constant pressure from our body weight as we move. As the stabilizing base to the lower extremities of our body, they are the critical foundation of our ability to maintain a healthy posture.

Posture is dependent not just on the structural components, but also on the unique sensory and reflex ability of the ankle and foot to maintain the critically important task of providing you with balance. Balance is made possible due to the specialized function of the ankle and foot in the sending and receiving of information to and from your brain and nervous system.

Your ankle and foot are intimately related and can be considered as a biomechanically connected unit or complex—working in tandem to ensure proper mobility. Podiatrists and orthopedists specializing in the foot and ankle are well aware of this ankle/foot relationship.

The workload of your ankle and foot is formidable. It is generally accepted that for every pound you weigh, your feet are exposed to triple that amount when you walk and seven times your body weight when you run. For example, if you weigh 200 pounds your feet absorb 600 pounds of force when you walk and 1,400 pounds of force when you run.

Due to this extreme pressure, an overwhelming majority of people experience some kind of painful foot/ankle condition at some point in their lives. Common causes of pain include ankle sprains, shin splints, arthritis, stress fractures, dropped arches, pronation, bunions, plantar fasciitis, hammertoes, heel spurs, and Tarsal Tunnel Syndrome.

A key to preventing the above conditions, as well as ankle and foot pain in general, is to gain a keen understanding of how the ankle and foot function together. Along with learning more about your ankles and feet to initiate a lifetime of pain-free, healthy movement, it is important to have a basic knowledge of appropriate footwear.

As a general rule, women's shoes tend to be more biomechanically detrimental for the delicate foot bones and mechanics of standing and walking than men's shoes. This is due to one major factor—unhealthy and constrictive designs. Men shoes tend to be roomier, with more support and low heels. Women's shoes, particularly with heels four inches or higher and a sharply pointed front, can cripple ankles and feet so badly that many podiatrists refer to this fashion for women as "shoe-icide."

High heels force the feet into an unnatural position that shifts the weight from the heel bone (the calcaneus, which is the largest of the tarsal or foot bones) to the much weaker toe bones (the metatarsal and phalangeal bones). Over time, high heels can lead to ankle weakness, swelling, stress fractures, and bony deformities such as bunions and hammertoes as well as shortening of the Achilles tendon to the point where the person has difficulty walking without heels.

Pointy toe shoes squeeze the front of your foot into an unnatural compressed tip and can cause bunions, blisters, corns, calluses, hammertoes, and lead to nerve pain—such as Morton's neuroma. At the other end of the spectrum are ballet flats, flip-flops and other shoes that offer no support. These are flimsy and can lead to plantar fasciitis due to the lack of arch support and shock absorber capabilities. Over time, these shoes can lead to a painful and potentially debilitating condition known as Tarsal Tunnel Syndrome.

You can prevent these painful conditions by wearing shoes with heels not higher than two inches with less pointed extremities or ones that slope to a point beyond your toes. Shoes made with a softer material as opposed to stiff leather can help. Whatever the shoe, make sure it has a strong shank and good arch support.

What about sneakers or those athletic shoes? The assumption is that they are the most ankle/foot-friendly shoes because they are designed to cushion and support for use in sports. While this is generally true, some high-end designers have included features such as extra supports and cushioning that can actually be detrimental to your ankles and feet. The key to wearing "healthy" sneakers appears to be the comfort you feel when you put them on. The greater the sense of comfort and support you feel, the greater the likelihood that you are wearing the sneakers that are right for you.

Another all too common and easily correctable cause of ankle and foot problems (as well as knee and hip) is that people, especially children, wear shoes that are the wrong size. This can lead to many foot problems, including arthritis. In the case of children, they can develop foot deformities as they mature. Parents often buy shoes a bit larger for their children to save money as they will "grow into them," or conversely, leave them in footwear that they have outgrown, perhaps trying to squeeze a little more mileage out of them. Both of these can lead to foot problems for children in the future.

The solution is to make sure that the length and width of your feet are measured correctly for every new pair of shoes using a Brannock Device®—the flat metal device that is available in most retail outlets that sell shoes. As your foot changes throughout your life, it is important to check the size and width each time you buy shoes.

THE ANKLE

Your ankle is composed of three bones: the tibia and fibula of the leg and the talus of the foot. The tibia (shin bone) forms the inner part of the ankle. The fibula (calf bone) forms the outer portion, and the talus (ankle bone) makes up the bottom part, which is where the ankle connects to the foot. The talus is cradled between the ends of the shin bone (medial malleolus) and calf bone (lateral malleolus) in what is commonly called the ankle mortise joint. The subtalar joint sits below the mortise joint and is comprised of the calcaneus (heel bone) and the talus.

The main muscles that govern the ankle include the calf muscles, the shin muscles and the muscles on the outer side of the ankle itself. The calf muscles are the main flexors of the ankle as you go up on your toes. The tibialis posterior muscle helps in flexion and also produces inversion, an inward motion of the foot, to stabilize the ankle joint. The tibialis posterior has a major role in maintaining the arches of the feet.

The shin muscle (tibialis anterior) brings the front of your foot upward and helps you to clear the ground as you walk. When this muscle becomes weak, people tend to trip over small elevations such as cracks in the sidewalk. This muscle also teams up with the tibialis posterior muscle to invert the foot and help support the medial arch of your foot.

The peroneal muscles are a group of muscles that support the outer part of your ankle and foot. These three muscles—the peroneus longus, peroneus brevis and peroneus tertius—are responsible for the outward motion or eversion of your ankle and foot. Keeping these muscles strong is a crucial factor in preventing ankle sprains.

The ankle is a hinge joint that predominately moves up (dorsiflexion) and down (plantarflexion). While it does move slightly side to side (inversion/eversion), it is not its primary function. It is important to note that the ankle is NOT a ball and socket joint and, therefore, does not rotate 360 degrees of motion naturally. While the ball and socket joints of the shoulder and hip can benefit from a circular stretch, the common practice found in dancing, martial arts and other exercise classes of *rotating* the ankle in a circle to warm it up can lead to a weakening of the ligaments around the ankle. Weakened ligaments are one of the principal causes of ankle sprains. Therefore, this well-meaning ritual of rotating the ankle as a "warm-up" should be discouraged.

The ligaments in the ankle are very susceptible to sprain, especially the anterior talofibular ligament (ATFL) on the outer part of your ankle which occurs with an *inversion* sprain when you "roll" your ankle. Eversion sprains are rare because the deltoid ligaments on the inside of your ankle are some of the most powerful ligaments in your body, plus the fact that the fibula extends lower on the outer part of the ankle than the tibia does on the inside—adding extra stability.

It is important to understand that any time you sprain your ankle, three injuries occur: the ankle bone (talus) slips out of alignment, the supporting muscles (peroneus group) are strained; and the surrounding ligaments are compromised or torn. All of these can impact the proper functioning of the ankle and foot and must be treated to ensure that they are functioning properly with each other. Too often, doctors treat the pain following a sprain with drugs and ankle wraps but don't take steps to realign the joint and strengthen the muscles that remain inhibited—this can lead to chronic ankle weakness and more serious problems.

Chronic flexing of the ankle due to high heel shoes, repeatedly stepping on the gas and brake pedals of a car or playing sports that require jumping can create a forward misalignment of the talus bone. Frequently, an ankle sprain will create a situation where your talus bone remains subluxated (slightly out of place) to the outer part of the joint and can lead to problems. Proper alignment of the ankle bone is critical to a strong and stable ankle/foot complex.

Along with the up-and-down movement of the foot at the ankle joint is the far subtler, but equally important, movement of shifting your weight from the three aspects of your foot: the hindfoot, midfoot, and forefoot. This movement is known as *translation*. Studies have shown that as people age, they lose this ability to efficiently translate their weight from one aspect of the foot to the other. It is believed that the loss of this ability, an integral aspect of what is known as position sense, is a common cause of falls in older persons. Position sense gives you the ability to shift your weight subconsciously and is critical in maintaining balance as well as preventing twisted ankles.

The Foot

Your foot is a delicate, supple structure meant to cushion every step you take and support your entire body as we move through our daily life. It is comprised of 26 bones, 33 joints, 107 ligaments, 19 muscles and tendons. In fact, the 52 bones in your feet make up about 25 percent of all the bones in your body. The foot has three arches (medial longitudinal, lateral longitudinal, anterior transverse) that connect and fan out to form a triangle. This triangle acts like a powerful trampoline to disperse the force of your body into the ground and respond by sending kinetic energy back up through you, giving a boost to your locomotion and a "bounce to your step."

The foot is unique in its ability to provide both mobility and stability when we walk—also known as the gait cycle. The gait cycle is comprised of the stance phase and the swing phase. The stance phase is when your foot is on the ground, and the swing phase is when it is moving forward in the air. The foot acts as a flexible shock absorber to cushion the jarring force of movement to your weight-bearing joints. It also provides strength and power to propel you forward and upward in walking and jumping.

Proper alignment of your ankle and foot bones allows them to send the correct signals to your brain to keep your reflexes sharp and your balance intact. Balancing exercises, including standing on a wobble board, specific yoga poses, shifting your weight forward/backward and side to side as you are standing in line at the store, or simply practicing balancing on one leg as you put your socks on, also contribute to a healthy position sense.

Conditions Associated with Ankle/Foot Problems

PEGGY, 45, had been working in an office since she was 18 years old. In keeping with the fashion trends and her workplace dress code, she wore high-heeled pointed shoes nearly every day for decades. Like many women, she had experienced foot pain and fatigue on and off for years. She developed bunions on the inside of both of her big toes. These bony structures made it difficult and painful to squeeze into high heels. Additionally, she found it harder to walk around barefoot at home because her heels tightened each time she tried. Both conditions had gotten so bad that she decided to see a podiatrist.

The podiatrist took X-rays and suggested that she needed surgery to remove the bunions and to lengthen the Achilles tendon that had shortened, due to years of wearing constrictive high-heels. She had heard horror stories from her female colleagues about bunion surgery. It's a painful procedure and takes weeks of recovery and physical therapy. The additional surgery to her Achilles tendon could extend the recovery period as well.

A friend and coworker related her own story of a painful bunion and Achilles tendon problem. A podiatrist suggested surgery, but the friend got a second opinion from her chiropractor who was certified in AK. After careful examination, she was able to avoid surgery by straightening out her bunion and lengthening her tendon. Now she could walk pain-free and learned to avoid wearing high heels whenever possible. Willing to try anything to relieve the pain and avoid surgery, Peggy made an appointment with this doctor.

As the consultation commenced, the doctor reviewed the X-rays taken by Peggy's podiatrist, which showed a bunion at the base of both big toes (metatarsophalangeal joint, also known as MTP) with a deviation of the toe out toward the second toe. This deviation is known as *hallux valgus* and is technically a subluxation of the big toe joint which causes it to press against the skin creating a bulge. If caught early enough, a doctor schooled in AK and chiropractic adjusting therapy can readily handle it. Occasionally, there may be bony overgrowth that can render the joint immobile and require surgery.

Postural Analysis revealed that Peggy stood with her weight forward on her toes and her knees slightly bent. Gait analysis showed that Peggy walked gingerly, leading with her toes. The doctor explained that the tightening in her Achilles tendon was essentially keeping her foot in an unnaturally pointed position, and this explained why she kept her knees bent when standing; namely to take pressure off of the tendon. This dysfunction contributed to her pain and bunions.

The doctor examined her feet and asked Peggy to straighten the big toe on each foot. While uncomfortable, she found that she was able to do it. The doctor gently manipulated the toes, without serious resistance from the bunions. This indicated that they had not fused with the bones yet. If the bunion, or subluxated toe, fuses within the joint, surgery is the only way to get rid of it. Peggy was relieved when the doctor told her the condition had not progressed to that point.

Muscle testing revealed gross weakness of the abductor hallicus muscle. This muscle runs the length of foot ending at the big toe and is essential in keeping the big toe straight and the arches functioning properly. Further examination using "pincer palpation", wherein the doctor gently squeezes the muscle/fascia, revealed a thickening of the fascia over the entire calf muscle—especially over the Achilles tendon. This tendon connects the calf muscles to the heel bone.

The initial diagnosis was that, due to years of walking in an unnatural position in restrictive high heels, the abductor hallicus muscle had become weakened, causing a misalignment of the metatarsophalangeal joint (MTP). This condition leads to stretching of the ligaments, inflammation of the soft tissues, and the buildup of calcified fibrous tissue or additional bone formation or *bunions*. Actually, much of Peggy's pain derived from Achilles tendonitis, a consequence of the thickening of the calf muscles. Fortunately, both conditions could be treated without any surgery.

Treatment began with a five-minute percussion of the MTP (bunion) using a Vibracussor® percussion device to gently release any fibrous and bony tissue that had accumulated in her foot. Afterward, a chiropractic adjustment was delivered to restore the big toe joints on both feet to their proper position. The doctor then performed spindle cell manipulation to stimulate the nerve endings in the abductor hallicus muscle to help facilitate the inhibited muscle and prepare it for rehabilitative exercises. Deep percussion therapy over various parts of the calf muscle relieved the tendon strain and inflammation.

The doctor gave Peggy two specific exercises to strengthen the abductor hallicus muscle. The first is called the "short foot exercise" where you sit and flex the muscles in the bottom of your foot between your heel and ball of the foot without flexing the toes. Hold the contraction for ten seconds and repeat for 7 repetitions. This exercise strengthens these weakened muscles and improves their ability to support the medial arch and the big toe. While doing this, you should feel your arch increase as you tighten the foot. The second exercise is to stand and curl your big toe into a carpet or rug. While maintaining this contraction, turn your heel inwards while squeezing the muscle on the inside of your foot that runs from your heel to your big toe. When you do this correctly, you will feel a tightening in this very neglected muscle. Hold this contraction for ten seconds and repeat seven times once a day.

Peggy required weekly treatments for 3 months to undo the years of damage from the chronic use of high-heeled pointed shoes. She was instructed not to wear high-heeled shoes during this time unless dictated by special occasions. She was able to find fashionable low-heeled shoes that fit the natural shape of her feet to wear daily. Peggy was diligent with her exercises and monthly treatments, and a year later her bunion had disappeared along with her foot pain.

* * *

JOHN, 18, enjoyed success as a star member of his high school long distance running team. In the summer before his freshman year in college, as he was training for the upcoming tryouts for the cross-country team, he severely twisted his left ankle. He went to the emergency room, where X-rays did not show a fracture, but his ankle was swollen, and he was in a great deal of pain. On the advice of his doctor and his coach, he treated it with rest, ice, over-the-counter anti-inflammatory drugs, Ace bandage compression, and elevation for two days. But the swelling did not go down, and the pain remained the same. With only a few weeks to go before he had to leave for college, John's parents suggested that he visit their Applied Kinesiologist. This individual had helped them with various conditions over the years, and they had great faith that he could shed some light on John's condition.

During his interview, John explained the circumstances of the accident and the nature of the pain he felt. He shared that before he twisted his ankle, he had begun to feel tightening in his left thigh as well as pain in his knee and hip when he walked.

Postural Analysis showed that John stood with his weight shifted onto his right side. Gait analysis revealed he limped more than walked and had to stop because of the pain in his foot and ankle. The Applied Kinesiologist observed that, in addition to the obvious limping, John's left foot was rolling inwards. This usually indicates instability of the ankle joint and a weakness of the outer ankle and foot muscles.

The doctor began the examination by asking John to remove the sneakers he was wearing. They showed considerable wear and tear on the outer part of the left shoe, especially at the heel. This indicated that John's weight was not distributed properly, causing him to put excessive pressure on the outer part of his left foot. As the shoe continued to wear, the improper weight distribution further shifted the strain to the outer part of the ankle. Over time, this could cause the ankle to become compromised and susceptible to sprain. It could also set off a chain reaction of misalignment upward to the knee and hip, causing additional pain.

The doctor placed a vibrating tuning fork over several bones of the ankle and foot. When John inquired about the procedure, the doctor said he was looking for fractures. John said that the X-rays in the emergency room didn't show any fractures. The Applied Kinesiologist explained that sometimes a small fracture might not show up for a few days in X-rays. The reason for this is that the break might be so slight that it goes undetected at first. When a vibrating tuning fork is placed directly over the injured bone, it will cause intense pain even if there is the slightest fracture because the outer part of the bone (periosteum) is rich in nerves. John said he only felt the vibration but no pain. Luckily, it confirmed that there was no fracture.

Functional muscle testing revealed inhibition of the peroneus muscles (longus and brevis) on the side of the ankle as well as a marked spasm of a hip muscle known as the tensor fasciae latae (TFL) muscle. This important muscle moves the thigh at the hip joint and stabilizes the knee by controlling the iliotibial (IT) band on the outer part of the thigh. The iliotibial band is made up of connective tissue known as fascia. It runs along the outer part of the thigh from the pelvis to the tibia and crosses both the hip and knee joints. The iliotibial band is an important stabilizing structure of the lateral (outer) part of the knee. In John's case, the IT band tightness came from its attempt to stabilize the outer part of the knee strained by the displaced ankle bone down below.

Based on these examination findings, the doctor concluded that John was suffering from displacement or subluxation of the talus, or ankle bone, due to the acute left ankle sprain. The sprain altered John's biomechanics of his left ankle and foot. He began to walk on the outside of left foot, causing the 5th metatarsal (pinky toe bone on the side of the foot) to slip down and essentially roll under his foot out of its normal alignment. As a consequence of these two misalignments, his ankle/foot complex signaled to his brain that it was unstable. This messaging forced the postural muscles to tighten involuntarily, causing pain in his knee and hip in addition to his ankle.

Treatment began with the doctor using the AK technique most effective in traumatic injuries, the Origin/Insertion Technique. He then applied percussion therapy, using the Vibracussor® and a gentle effleurage massage technique to reduce some of the swelling around the ankle. The doctor also used percussion therapy to release the fascial thickening encasing the TFL muscle and the IT band.

The AK practitioner then utilized precise chiropractic adjustive therapy to realign the side of the foot (fifth metatarsal), ankle bone (talus), and the secondary knee bone (fibula) that also makes up the outer part of the ankle joint. John experienced immediate relief from the pain and swelling.

After John's foot, ankle and knee bones were properly aligned, the doctor carefully placed two strips of athletic tape under the pinky toe to stabilize it. He gave John a specific exercise to simultaneously strengthen the peroneus muscles and the TFL to prevent future ankle sprains and to stabilize the knee and hip joints.

Also, John had to wear a soft knee and ankle brace and begin some light running exercises so his muscles could get used to the proper alignments of his ankle, foot, knee, and hip. He was told to use a foam roller to massage the fascia of his outer leg muscles (IT band) to help relieve any tightness. The doctor recommended that John get new sneakers as well. The patient returned for several additional treatments to ensure the alignment and healing process.

On the third visit, the doctor noticed that while the healing process was proceeding well, it could benefit from some *proprioceptive neuromuscular facilitation* exercises (PNF) whereby the doctor provides resistance and John moves his ankle diagonally up and in, then down and out for two sets of 12 repetitions. These PNF resistance stretches increase the flexibility and muscular strength of the ankle and help with the healing process, along with aiding in the prevention of future injury.

On the fourth visit, John reported that he had a severe setback, and the pain returned. This setback seemed odd to his doctor until John mentioned that it happened after he had put on a new pair of running shoes to break them in. He had brought them along for the doctor to examine. The new shoes were a different brand from his original sneaker and had some design features that had thrown his bones out of alignment. The doctor suggested that John try a new pair of shoes from the same company. After a new alignment and some light running exercises in the new shoes, the pain disappeared; John was able to resume his usual training regimen. He made the college team and returns for check-ups when he comes back home.

* * *

DENISE, 32, was a waitress with dreams of becoming an actress. She ran around New York City, attending acting classes and auditions during the day and working long shifts at a restaurant at night. Gradually, she noticed soreness in both of her feet that she attributed to her grueling schedule of standing and walking for nearly sixteen hours a day. She tried using generic orthotic pads in her shoes, soaking her feet at night, and sitting more often. Nothing helped. The soreness developed into a sharp, stabbing pain in the bottom of her feet that forced her to miss work and auditions.

She went to a podiatrist, who said that she had an excessive pronation problem. Pronation is a normal side-to-side motion of the foot, whereby the arches move to provide shock absorption and adaptation to uneven surfaces. Excessive pronation occurs when the foot rolls inwards and the arches "flatten," compromising their cushioning function. The condition is commonly known as "flat feet" and can lead to any number of painful conditions including foot and ankle pain, plantar fasciitis, bunions, Morton's neuroma, hammer toes, heel spurs, Tarsal Tunnel Syndrome, as well as knee, hip, low back, and even neck and jaw pain.

It is a common misconception that "flat feet" are genetic in nature. While some people may have an inherited trait that may contribute to a propensity to have dropped arches (medically known as pes planus), it is more likely that this condition is caused by a variety of environmental factors such as poor diet, lack of proper muscle function usually due to stress which instinctively leads people to place too much weight on their toes, inadequate footwear, weak foot muscles, and poor posture.

The podiatrist prescribed customized hard orthotic inserts for Denise's shoes. Orthotics provide additional support to keep the arches in position. As helpful as they can be, they only treat the symptoms of excessive pronation, not the cause. After several weeks, Denise's pain did not get any better. Late one night at the restaurant, a coworker saw her crying in the corner of the restaurant while rubbing her feet. He asked her what was wrong, and she shared her situation with him. He said that he suffered from the same condition and received the same treatment from the first podiatrist he visited. But it wasn't until he visited a podiatrist who was also certified in AK that he finally found the relief he needed. Willing to try anything, she agreed to see his doctor.

After an in-depth consultation and inspection of the hard-orthotic inserts, the doctor agreed with the initial diagnosis of Denise's podiatrist. However, after removing the orthotics, the doctor also examined the shoes she was wearing. They were severely lacking in arch support and could be a contributing factor to her pain. The hard orthotics were designed to compensate for this lack of support. However, hard orthotics work similar to putting your foot into a cast; since they never allow the muscles that support the arch to strengthen, they can exacerbate the problem. Postural Analysis revealed two classic indicators of excessive pronation:

Helbing's sign, wherein the tendon that connects the calf muscle to the heel (the Achilles tendon) curves inwards, and a flattening of one of the longitudinal arches in each foot. In other words, while Denise was standing, the doctor could see her feet "flattening out" and drastically losing their shock absorber capabilities. Gait Analysis confirmed a dramatic collapsing of the arch when Denise walked.

The examination progressed to the muscle-testing portion. The doctor began with what is called the Shock Absorber Challenge. This is a procedure unique to AK, whereby the doctor administers pressure with a closed fist to the bottom of the feet. Denise felt the same pain as if she were walking or standing. Further muscle testing revealed that the tibialis posterior muscles in both feet were inhibited. This muscle is critical to maintaining the integrity of the ankle joint as well as the arches, especially when walking.

Finally, the doctor found that one of the tarsal bones, specifically the navicular, in the arches of both feet had become misaligned and had dropped down. This bone forms the top of your arches when it is in its proper position and maintains the integrity of the arches along with a network of ligaments. When the ligaments are compromised, the navicular bone moves out of position, and the arch can drop—causing excessive pronation.

The doctor explained that Denise's condition was complex but eminently treatable. The podiatrist began treatment by adjusting the navicular bone in each foot, using an Arthrostim® tool. This specialized device utilizes a high-speed thrust and recoil motion that allows your doctor to gently make an accurate mechanical correction to a troubled joint. Through the precise realignment of the navicular bone into its proper position at the apex of the arch, it helps to correct several foot joints that provide the flexibility of the foot during walking. Denise's doctor also employed the Origin/Insertion Technique to facilitate the weakened tibialis posterior muscles to help maintain the proper position of the navicular bone, specifically, and the arches in general.

After making the necessary corrections to the bones and muscles, the doctor then took a mold for soft orthotic inserts designed specifically for her *now properly aligned feet.* Soft orthotics are less expensive than the hard variety and can often be prepared in the doctor's office. They are flexible and allow the muscles of the feet to strengthen more naturally than the harder version. They were ready in a short time while Denise waited.

Before leaving, the doctor gave Denise a guide to proper posture. Proper posture aids in healthy weight distribution and is essential to preventing dropped arches. Your weight should be distributed evenly throughout the entire foot, predominately centered over the large heel bone (calcaneus). Putting too much weight over your toes will fatigue the ligaments and muscles and compromise your arch, causing the foot to eventually drop and excessively pronate. The doctor also gave Denise a bottle of low-dose manganese. Manganese is necessary for ligament strength, which will, in turn, help support the arches. The podiatrist also suggested that Denise include more foods high in manganese in her diet including blueberries, beets, mussels, tea, whole grains, leafy vegetables, nuts, and seeds. Also, the doctor suggested several different brands of sneakers that would give Denise better support than the shoes that she was wearing. Finally, the doctor suggested that she try to adjust her schedule to allow her damaged muscles to heal.

Denise returned in two weeks and happily reported that her feet felt immensely better. Due to the lack of pain, she had less stress and more energy than ever.

* * *

DOMENICK was an 80-year-old retired firefighter. A big, muscular man, he had been used to a wide variety of physical challenges during his 26 years of fighting fires. So, when he started experiencing severe pain in the bottom of his left foot, specifically in the back of his heel, he just wrote it off and hoped that it would pass. However, after four months it had gotten so bad that he found it impossible to walk without limping. He visited a podiatrist and had X-rays taken. He received a diagnosis of plantar fasciitis and the beginnings of a heel spur.

Plantar fasciitis is a condition that results from the inflammation of the plantar muscles located on the bottom of your feet. A heel spur is a calcium deposit that causes a bony protrusion, usually on the underside of the heel where the tendon of the plantar muscles connects to the heel bone. Both of these conditions often occur together and are extremely painful.

The podiatrist suggested a cortisone shot to relieve the pain, soaking the foot in warm water and Epsom salts, and special orthotics that would help the foot heal. Domenick took the shot and began soaking his feet daily but decided to pass on the expensive custom-made orthotics and bought generic foot pads from the drugstore instead. However, after a short period of relief, his pain came back. It was particularly acute when he climbed the stairs in his home.

His daughter recommended that he get another opinion and suggested that he see her podiatrist, who was also certified in AK. He had helped relieve a painful condition in her arch without special orthotics or shots. Domenick agreed.

During the initial interview, Domenick explained his problem and shared with the doctor the X-rays, diagnosis, and treatments he had received from the first podiatrist. He reported that there had been no recent injury to the foot and started to notice a problem walking after climbing the stairs multiple times to put Christmas decorations back into the attic. The pain started as a dull ache and gradually progressed to the severe sharp pain he had been suffering with for the past four months.

After reviewing the X-rays, the AK specialist agreed with the first podiatrist's diagnosis of plantar fasciitis and the beginnings of a heel spur. Postural Analysis revealed that Domenick stood with his weight shifted predominately onto his right foot. On Gait Analysis, he walked with a distinct limp, obviously trying to keep as much pressure off his left foot as possible when it touched the ground. Recently, he had started using a cane but did not bring it with him to the appointment.

The examination then progressed to the muscle-testing portion. Muscle testing revealed three important clues: a strain of Domenick's plantar muscles; a shortening of the fascia of the calf or gastrocnemius muscle, which helps to hold the heel bone in place; and a weakness of one of the muscles that helps bend the big toe (flexor hallicus brevis) as you push off the ground when you walk, especially when climbing stairs.

The Applied Kinesiologist explained to Domenick that when we walk, we employ a heel to toe motion. However, when we climb stairs, we rely heavily on our toes. In Domenick's case, going up the stairs to the attic repeatedly caused his calf muscles to tighten and to pull the heel bone back, unnaturally forcing it out of alignment. Over time, the displacement of the heel compromised ligaments surrounding the tarsal tunnel and led to impingement on the nerve that runs through it, causing pain and the flexor muscle in his toe to become inhibited. This is a common condition when you walk upstairs frequently. However, in most cases, walking normally after climbing will inadvertently realign your heel bone before symptoms occur due to the natural motion of landing on your heel then shifting your weight to your toes. This tends to *knock* your heel bone back into alignment. Unfortunately, this did not happen in Dominick's case, and the chronic backward displacement of his heel also strained the plantar muscles, causing his plantar fasciitis and the buildup of calcium on the heel to create a spur and additional pain.

Plantar fasciitis, toe weakness and the beginnings of a heel spur are all consistent findings of someone suffering from *Tarsal Tunnel Syndrome*. This is similar to Carpal Tunnel Syndrome (CTS) in the hand, except that this involves pinching of the tibial nerve that runs between the tarsal bones in the foot. Like CTS, Tarsal Tunnel Syndrome can lead to muscle weakness and eventually to a deformity in the feet known as *hammertoes*. Domenick was suffering from Tarsal Tunnel Syndrome but luckily not long enough for a hammertoe deformity to develop.

Knowing the precise cause of his conditions, the doctor began treatment with an AK medical massage technique to lengthen the shortened fascial covering over the calf muscles through deep percussion therapy with a Vibracussor®. He used Origin/Insertion Technique to facilitate the injured plantar muscles. Finally, he restored the heel bone to its proper forward position, using an Arthrostim® adjusting tool. While Domenick still felt pain, he related that some of the sharpest pain in the bottom of his heel and strain in his calf were greatly relieved.

After the first treatment, Domenick was instructed to gently tap his bare heel at home on a carpeted floor several times a day to ensure its proper alignment. Since he needed to climb stairs in his home, the doctor showed him how to walk upstairs sideways to avoid using his toes until he was fully healed.

The doctor gave Domenick calf stretches and taught him how to pick up a towel with his toes by contracting his foot muscles. These two exercises done in conjunction and repeated several times a day helped to loosen his tight fascia encasing the calf muscles and strengthen his plantar muscles. Domenick was also instructed to roll his foot over a tennis ball to help relieve the heel spur pain and keep the plantar muscles supple. Finally, the doctor then fitted him for a soft orthotic to help maintain the bones in the feet in their proper position while also helping to strengthen the plantar muscles. After ten treatments over the next few months, Domenick's condition had completely disappeared. On a follow-up visit a year later, an X-ray revealed that the heel spur had been reabsorbed and was now gone.

* * *

It is well known that for every action there is a reaction. This is true of our body's ability to act and react to imbalances. It is important to address the body's capacity to adapt to and compensate for both acute injuries and chronic stress. Unfortunately, traditional medicine's approach of focusing on the symptoms can sometimes become so specialized that it neglects the true source of the problem. Perhaps nowhere is the incredible relationship of seemingly non-related parts of your body more apparent than in the ankle/foot complex. Something as simple as poor shoe choices and a manganese-deficient diet can lead to problems that affect the proper mobility of your entire body.

Action and reaction. Cause and effect. Balance and imbalance. Nearly every instance of dysfunction in the body will result in symptoms that require an in-depth investigation to find and cure the underlying problem, no matter where it might be. The art and science of AK strives to help your doctor to differentiate between the symptoms you feel and the actual source of the problem, no matter how counterintuitive it may be. Precise diagnosis and appropriate treatment are principal factors in everyone's personal health equation.

8

LOW BACK PAIN

Do you know what the #1 disability is in the world? If you guessed low back pain, you would be right. According to *Annals of the Rheumatic Diseases*, recent studies report that "Low back pain (LBP) causes more disability globally than any other condition...." As the world population continues to age, an urgent need exists for research to find out why and how LBP might be prevented or better managed."[20] Eighty percent of adults experience low back pain at some point in their life.

Low back pain comprises a full spectrum of symptoms, ranging from experiencing stiffness when getting up out of bed in the morning, to the aches and pains from sitting too long or exercising, to the paralyzing muscle spasms and searing pain that radiates down the leg. Just as the range of symptoms is diverse, so are the conditions that contribute to it. Age, trauma, prolonged sitting, and improper lifting habits are just a few of the possible causes. In fact, some of the sources of the pain don't even originate in the low back itself. AK is uniquely positioned to find the actual causes of the painful symptoms, offering both relief and ongoing health without radical intervention such as surgery.

The Low Back

Your low back is the connecting point between the torso and the pelvis. It is what allows you to bend, lift, swing, throw, walk, and run. Essentially, it comprises the lumbar spine, which is located just beneath the thoracic spine in the middle of the back, the sacrum bone, the pelvic bones, and the musculature that surrounds them.

The lumbar spine is made up of five vertebrae (spinal bones). These are the largest of the spinal vertebrae and are responsible for supporting the entire spine, as well as the weight of your upper body. They curve forward in a concave position toward the abdominal muscles. This curvature is known as lordosis and gives your low back the ability to support the pressures of your upper body weight while providing the flexibility and mobility necessary for nearly every motion we perform.

Separating each vertebra is a fibrocartilage disc which serves as a sort of shock absorber and cushion to prevent compression of the vertebrae. Your intervertebral discs are responsible for 25% of your spinal height. When you consider that the average adult spine is approximately 24 to 28 inches in length, this means that your fully hydrated discs comprise six to seven of those inches. Loss of disc height results when people do not properly care for their spines with chiropractic or osteopathic treatments and adequate water intake. Generally, it is the principal reason why people *shrink* dramatically as they age.

Each disc consists of a tough outer wall called the annulus fibrous and a gelatinous inner section known as the nucleus pulposus. Unlike many bone and cartilage structures in the body, blood does not flow through spinal discs. Instead, the discs rely upon a mechanical process known as an *imbibing pump* that allows the free flow of nutrients into the disc and the drainage of metabolic waste, primarily lactic acid, out of it. This "pump" is dependent upon the unrestricted movement of the vertebral bones above and below the disc. A restriction of proper spinal bone motion disrupts this complicated osmotic transfer of fluid between the inside of your disc and the surrounding area, resulting in a weakening of the disc due to lack of nutrients and a buildup of waste. The extra waste can cause the disc to swell, creating increased pressure on the nerve.

When there is weakness or injury of the disc, the external wall can be damaged, and the inner gel-like portion exudes, effectively removing the cushion between vertebrae and causing pressure on the nerve that passes through them. This condition is known as a disc herniation. Disc herniation, while not commonly a factor in most lower back problems, is one of the chief causes in cases of severe low back and leg pain. It is usually preceded or accompanied by a restriction in the movement of the spinal bones (known as spinal fixations) or a slight misalignment of the spinal bones (known as spinal subluxations), which disrupt the biomechanics of the spine and compromise the disc. Thirty-one pairs of nerves exit the central spinal cord at spaces in and between the vertebrae, known as intervertebral foramen. The nerves in the lower back include the five lumbar and sacral nerves and one pair of coccygeal nerves. Several of the lumbar and sacral nerves combine to form the sciatic nerve, which is the largest nerve in your body. These nerves control or contribute to the function of your lower back, hips, bladder, intestines, legs, and sex organs.

In addition to the lumbar spine and discs, the bones of the pelvis are crucial to the overall functioning of the low back. This complex of bones includes the right and left ilium, right and left ischium, and the central sacrum which connects directly to the lumbar vertebrae. The ilium forms a large crest on each side of the pelvis, extending down to become the ischia or "butt bones" in the rear. The sacrum is located at the bottom of the lumbar spine and is actually five bones fused into one. It is a triangular shaped structure with the point facing downward. At the bottom of the point is the tiny coccyx or "tail" bone.

The muscles of the lower back and pelvis are crucial to the protection and proper function of the lumbar spine and pelvis. The principal muscles of the low back include the paraspinal muscles that run along your spinal column; the psoas muscles that connect the hip to all five of your lumbar vertebrae, including the discs themselves; the quadratus lumborum that connect from the pelvic bone to the 12th rib; the abdominals that stabilize the spine and support the abdominal organs, especially the intestines, bladder and uterus; the gluteal and piriformis muscles in the buttocks area; and the adductor muscles in the groin region. All of these muscles, when functioning properly, provide your low back with strength, flexibility, and stability. Weak or compromised muscles in this region often lead to improper alignment of the vertebrae, which contributes to disc herniation and low back pain.

While not generally considered part of the low back musculature, several muscles are intimately related to low back function because they connect to the pelvis. Included in this group are two large muscles—the sartorius (the longest muscle in your body) running from the top of the pelvis to the inner part of your knee, and the latissimus dorsi (the widest muscle in your body) extending from the pelvis and low back up to the shoulder.

Like nearly every other structure of our bodies, the low back works synergistically with our entire skeletal and muscular system to allow us to move freely. Any imbalance in the low back complex can lead to a variety of life-altering conditions such as muscle spasms, strains, or weaknesses; scoliosis (unhealthy curvature of the spine); stenosis (narrowing of the spinal column); herniated discs; sciatica (burning low back and leg pain); piriformis syndrome (spasm of the butt muscle); subluxations (misalignments of vertebrae and bone structures); and spinal fixations (a locking up of the vertebrae).

The main cause of many of these conditions can be traced back to some kind of misalignment of the bones in the low back region in conjunction with a dysfunction of the surrounding muscles. Functional muscle testing pinpoints the imbalance. Applied Kinesiology techniques treat these conditions effectively and help prevent future injuries to the bones, muscles, and discs through a unique combination of spinal adjustment and muscle manipulation, supported by strengthening or flexibility exercises and nutrition.

Conditions Associated with Low Back Pain

HENRY, 35, was a successful high school football coach. Before he started his coaching career, he had played college football and injured his low back. Like many athletes, he fluffed it off at the time and just worked through the pain. But the pain never went away and got progressively worse over the years. He had tried orthopedic, chiropractic and osteopathic doctors, physical therapists, cortisone shots, and both prescription and over-the-counter pain medications. While he got temporary relief from many of these treatments, the pain always came back. However, none of these specialists ever diagnosed its cause. Eventually, it had gotten so bad that it was starting to affect his ability to coach his players.

One of his team assistants told Henry about a new sports injury clinic that had just opened nearby. Henry had been to so many similar clinics that it hardly seemed like news. However, he learned that this clinic was different; the doctors there incorporated AK into their therapies. According to the assistant, this specialty worked wonders on any kind of sports-related pain. Willing to try anything at this point, Henry made an appointment.

Henry arrived at the clinic in so much pain that he filled out the patient profile leaning over the front desk since it alleviated some of his back pain.

During the initial consultation, Henry had to stand with both arms on the back of a chair as he related his history to the doctor. Until recently, he said that he had always been able to cope with the pain and hide it from everyone, especially his players; but it had gotten so bad that he had a hard time keeping up appearances. He was beginning to miss practices, which could jeopardize his team and his job. He lost sleep and was generally miserable. The doctor dug deeper and asked Henry exactly what happened when he had injured his low back as a young man. Henry related, "I went to block someone who was much bigger, and when we collided, the pain exploded in my lower back."

After making a note of this incident of spinal compression, the doctor reviewed his medical records and X-rays. They confirmed the doctor's suspicions. The X-rays revealed a misalignment of the Hadley's S Curve in his low back region. This meant that Henry was suffering from jamming of his lumbar vertebrae. This jamming created an accentuated and painful curve in his spine (hyperlordosis) that compromised its function. The normal configuration of the joints (known as facets) of the lumbar spine that connect the vertebrae forms an "S" shape. If there is an abrupt interruption or "break" in the smooth contour of this "S" configuration, this means that the lumbar vertebrae have become jammed together in a condition known as *facet imbrication.*

The doctor pointed out the problem on the X-ray to Henry. "It looks like this is where you got jammed up in college and have been dealing with it ever since."

Henry was shocked. "If it's been like this for years, why didn't the other doctors see it on the X-rays?"

"Actually, they probably did. However, most likely, they were looking for a serious fracture instead of a misalignment, so it's easy to miss. The acute inflammation around the injury masks it as well. I'll need to do a physical examination to confirm the condition."

Postural Analysis showed Henry leaning over slightly to his right, almost as if he was carrying a weight on his right shoulder. Gait analysis revealed that Henry walked with a distinct disparity between his legs. His right foot hit the ground with far more force than the left. The sound was so distinct that it actually sounded like Henry was wearing a sneaker on the left foot and a hard-heeled heavy boot on the right—he was wearing sneakers on both feet.

The examination began with an orthopedic test known as Kemp's test, wherein the patient is asked to lean back while bending and twisting to one side and then the other to see if there is any pain in the low back and/or down the leg. When Henry moved to the right, he experienced a sharp pain in his low back, as well as pain radiating down into the back of his right thigh. Then the doctor had Henry lie on the examination table face up with one leg bent while he applied traction to the other leg with a gentle, yet quick pull. If the extended leg becomes inhibited, it indicates facet imbrication. Henry tested positive for a facet imbrication on his right side.

The examination progressed to the muscle-testing portion, which revealed inhibition of the quadratus lumborum (QL) muscle on the left, causing a tightening of the QL muscle on the right. *Applied Kinesiological research has discovered that the physiological inhibition of one muscle often results in the spasm of a related muscle.*

While many therapies do an excellent job of finding and treating the muscle spasm, they often neglect treating related muscles that may be inhibited as well. Without treating *all* the compromised muscles, the condition will persist.

After the examination, the doctor diagnosed Henry with facet imbrication, which had begun with his initial incident in college. He had strained his left QL and jammed the right side of his lumbar spine. The strain on the left caused a spasm in the right QL. As it was left untreated for over a decade, the spasm kept the lumbar vertebrae jammed into each other, causing spinal compression and constant pain. This would also explain why leaning over the reception desk alleviated some of his pain—Henry was unconsciously unjamming his compressed low back.

The AK treatment which is usually indicated in cases of low back physical trauma begins with the application of the Origin/Insertion technique to stimulate the inhibited muscles into proper function. A medical massage technique known as Fascial Release helps to "iron out" or lengthen the shortened fascia of the subsequent muscle spasm to restore the normal fascia/muscle relationship. In Henry's case, Origin/Insertion Technique was administered to the left QL muscle, and fascial release was applied to the right QL muscle.

After balancing out the muscles, the doctor restored the lumbar spine back to proper alignment. He had Henry lie on his back with his left leg bent upright at the knee. The doctor then applied traction to the extended right thigh twenty times until he felt a release in pressure. Essentially, the doctor "unjammed" the low back. When Henry got off the examination table and stood, he couldn't believe it. The pain that he had lived with for over a decade was barely noticeable.

The doctor gave Henry several simple exercises to do at home. Each morning and each evening, he needed to lie on his back and bring his knees to his chest and hold it for thirty seconds. He also told him to hang from a chinning bar at the conclusion of every day. During his usual gym workout, he needed to avoid squats with any weight on his shoulders, arching his back in a "backbend stretch," and jumping down from a step to hit the ground hard.

These actions put undue pressure on the lumbar spine and could cause a relapse.

Henry required just four more treatments to ensure that the muscles were balanced, and the vertebrae were no longer jammed together. He diligently did his knee/chest stretches and avoided the exercises where weights could compress his spine. Henry could hardly believe his back pain was finally gone—he felt like he had a new lease of life.

* * *

KAREN, 40, was a pediatrician who was suffering from low back pain and numbness, muscle cramps and a sharp pain radiating down her legs for almost three years. At first, it was manageable and, not unlike many doctors with a busy practice, she didn't make the time to take care of her own problem. She simply relied on over-the-counter drugs and hot baths. However, over time, the pain had become so severe that she could hardly stand or lean over to examine her little patients or sit to consult with their parents. She couldn't get a good night's sleep. Since she could not sit for any length of time without pain, she had to rent a van to lie down in while someone else drove her to her office.

She visited a colleague of hers, an orthopedic surgeon. After viewing her X-rays and MRI, he diagnosed her with spinal stenosis. Spinal stenosis is a condition in which the lumbar vertebrae are compressed, causing an abnormal narrowing of the spinal canal that surrounds the nerves in the spinal cord. This narrowing creates pressure on the nerve, resulting in severe pain in the low back and often the legs.

Due to the severity of her problem, Karen's friend recommended the orthodox medical treatment for this condition: laminectomy. A laminectomy is a surgical procedure performed on the low back where the lamina, the portion of the spinal bone that forms the vertebral arch that surrounds your lumbar spinal cord, is removed to relieve the pressure on the nerve roots that exit between the bones. Given the escalating nature of her pain, he believed this procedure to be the most appropriate cure for her stenosis.

Despite the risks, Karen was considering this option when the unexpected good news arrived that she was pregnant. She immediately stopped the over-the-counter pain medication she had been taking. Additionally, she and her doctors agreed upon the decision to postpone the surgery and wait until after she gave birth to avoid any danger to the baby. However, her pain was worse than ever, and she began to worry about her general physical and emotional health and their effects on her baby. What could she do about the pain for the next nine months? Her options seemed to have run out.

Then her cousin, who had been diagnosed by two orthopedic surgeons with a lumbar disc herniation, told Karen about a doctor of chiropractic specializing in AK who had helped her with her severe low back pain. Both surgeons had recommended she undergo surgery as well. Knowing the risks of any spinal surgery, her cousin sought a third opinion. A friend recommended her doctor "who worked miracles" with low back pain. The cousin took the recommendation and was cured of her condition without surgery. Karen was skeptical of this nontraditional approach but agreed to meet with him.

At the initial consult, the doctor reviewed the X-rays, CT, MRI and Electromyography (EMG) reports of her low back and legs. While he agreed with the general diagnosis of some level of pressure on the spinal nerve, he was not certain that it was due to stenosis. There was a slight narrowing of the spinal canal, but nothing dramatic enough to produce the kind of pain she experienced. There was no indication of bone spurs at the foramina (the hole where the nerve root exits the spinal cord) either, which are commonly associated with the leg pain and cramping. However, the severity of Karen's pain led him to believe there might be some other condition causing it.

He explained to her that doctors of chiropractic and osteopathy have long asserted that low back pain can be traced to some kind of misalignment or restriction of movement of the bones in the lumbar spine. Misalignments cause inflammation, muscle spasms, and joint degeneration and lead to improper nerve impulses, resulting in pain. Most of these conditions can be remedied with precise spinal adjustments and treatment of the muscles surrounding the area.

Occasionally, due to degenerative changes or severe trauma, the bone might be fractured and might need to be removed. However, this was not the case for Karen. Doctors of chiropractic and osteopathy feel that it makes more sense to apply precise spinal adjustive therapy first before considering any kind of surgery in this sensitive region of the body.

Needless to say, Karen was relieved to hear that she might not need surgery after all.

The AK specialist pursued his examination. Gait Analysis revealed that Karen barely extended either of her legs behind her as she walked so that she almost waddled as she moved forward. Postural Analysis revealed an excessive curve in the lumbar region (hyperlordosis). Muscle testing revealed inhibition of the gluteus maximus muscles on both sides. The gluteus maximus helps the proper function of your legs and stabilizes the pelvis (specifically, the ilium), and prevents it from slipping forward.

Further AK testing using the Joint Challenge revealed that Karen's fifth lumbar vertebra, along with both ilia bones of the pelvis, had become misaligned; this could explain the spinal stenosis-like symptoms of low back and leg pain.

Lastly, the AK examination revealed a cranio-cervical syndrome, or restriction of the flow of cerebrospinal fluid (CSF) throughout the entire spine due to a slight dysfunction in the rhythmic motions of the skull. The spinal fluid flows from inside the brain down the entire spinal cord through subtle motions of the skull. CSF cushions, protects, and nourishes the brain, spinal cord and the nerve roots that exit the spinal cord. Any interruption of this flow could cause pain anywhere in the body, and very commonly in the lower extremities—particularly in the low back and legs.

The Applied Kinesiologist rendered an initial diagnosis of subluxations (misalignments) of the lumbar spine and ilium bones as well as cranio-cervical syndrome. The doctor explained to Karen that the chronic lack of skull movement (probably from jaw clenching and tension due to stress) and misalignments of her spine and pelvis compromised the integrity of lumbar spinal nerves. Most traditional orthopedic surgeons diagnose it as stenosis and recommend surgery, but in Karen's case, the actual cause of the problem was not the lamina bone but a combination of misalignment, muscle weakness, and poor spinal fluid distribution.

As a medical doctor, Karen had a difficult time understanding this diagnosis. She'd never heard of cranio-cervical syndrome and found it difficult to accept that it could contribute to the intense pain she had in her low back and legs. Her medical training never mentioned that the skull moved at all or had any relationship with spinal fluid. She also couldn't understand what had caused such a serious misalignment in her lumbar and pelvic region.

The Applied Kinesiologist explained that research showed that the bones comprising the skull, along with the mandible (jaw bone), are in subtle reciprocal motion all the time and contribute to the flow of spinal fluid. The sutures that are between the cranial bones can be considered the intervertebral discs of the skull in that they allow for compression and tension release along with the subtle motion of your skull. When this motion was restricted, it affected the CSF flow and the nerves along the spine straight down to the lumbar region. Together with the lumbar and pelvic misalignments, probably caused by repetitive movements such as lifting babies all day with extended sitting and bending over an examination table, it was a recipe for her chronic pain.

Karen thought for a while about the logic of the Applied Kinesiologist's explanation. Still not fully convinced, she asked how he would treat the condition.

He explained that the treatment consisted of chiropractic adjustive therapy to restore normal alignment of the lumbar and pelvic bones to improve the function of the primary motor nerve that supplies the gluteus maximus muscle so it could function properly. Then he would perform a gentle manipulation of the skull bones to restore its normal motion.

Karen agreed to give it a try.

After the doctor was finished with the first treatment session, Karen let out a deep sigh of relief. It was the first time in over three years that her pain diminished. She could sit and walk without wincing. It did, indeed, seem like a miracle. And the best part was that it appeared that she could avoid surgery if the treatment lasted.

Karen required a total of twelve treatments to stabilize the region fully. To reinforce the adjustments, the doctor gave her a sacroiliac belt to wear over her pelvis, as well as stretching exercises for the low back and strengthening exercises for her gluteus maximus muscles. Karen was also taught how to protect her lower back by bending over at the hips instead of bending at the spine. Bending at the hips—also known as *hip hinging*—takes pressure off the back muscles by engaging the gluteus maximus and hamstrings muscles, thus keeping the back straight like a table. She was also encouraged to do deep breathing exercises and meditation to help with stress reduction and maintain the corrections to her cranium and CSF flow.

During her treatment, Karen was given natural anti-inflammatory supplements that are safe to take during pregnancy such as omega 3 oils, trace minerals, B vitamins, and especially zinc and magnesium. Omega 3 oils, along with these cofactor nutrients, are particularly important, as they help to create prostaglandins 1 and 3—our body's natural anti-inflammatories. Karen went on to a full recovery and was healthy enough to add the demanding job of motherhood to her busy pediatric practice.

* * *

LUKE, 28, was a highly successful salesman. He spent long hours visiting accounts, sitting in meetings with clients, and driving throughout his sales territory. One morning, he woke up with severe low back pain that pierced through his right buttocks and down his right leg. He never had this kind of pain before. He had always enjoyed good health, ate wisely, and exercised. He had a busy schedule that day, so he took a few over-the-counter pain suppressants and tried to cope with it. However, as the day progressed, the pain worsened whenever he was in a sitting position. Driving was particularly difficult. That night, the pain prevented him from sleeping. He tried more over-the-counter medication, but it upset his stomach.

After a few days of agony, he then went to a chiropractor for relief, but inexplicably his condition worsened after the visit. Over the next few weeks, he had to cut back on his work schedule and was forced to service many of his clients by phone instead of in person. Both his social and professional lives suffered. He became depressed, which made matters worse. Finally, he visited two highly regarded back specialists, one being an orthopedist and the other a neurosurgeon, and had a full range of X-rays and MRI's done.

The films indicated two severely herniated discs in the lumbar region. Both specialists recommended back surgery; one recommended a laminectomy and the other a spinal fusion procedure where the doctor would insert bone grafts using titanium rods and screws to connect them to the spine. Luke was concerned, not only about what he had heard about the risks of back surgery but also about the 6–8 weeks it would take to recover. He couldn't afford to miss so much time from work. Luke didn't know what to do. Meanwhile, his pain continued.

One day during a sales visit to a long-time client, Luke couldn't hide his discomfort and apologized for having to stand during their meeting. The client recommended that he visit his chiropractor. Luke shuddered at the suggestion, as his past experience with chiropractic was not positive. He thanked his client and took the doctor's number with no intention of calling. Sensing his reluctance, the client told Luke that this doctor was not only a skilled chiropractor but was also certified in AK, a specialty that heals many serious conditions without surgery or drugs. The doctor had helped him and many of his friends with a wide variety of painful conditions. Having nothing to lose, Luke agreed to make an appointment for another opinion.

During the consultation, Luke had to stand because of the pain. He shared that the pain he had been suffering with for several months seemed to have come out of nowhere. He hadn't fallen or lifted anything heavy or had any other traumatic event that would explain it. He loved his sales job, even though it had him on the road up to 14 hours a day. Now, it was in jeopardy as he could hardly drive short distances or sit with clients. The doctor listened intently and took notes.

The doctor asked him to describe his business day. Luke said that he would begin with prearranged sales meetings with his clients, for which he would carry a special backpack filled with sample products. After his sales visits, he would spend hours on the phone following up, often walking and talking as he commuted home.

The orthopedic, neurological X-ray, and MRI reports that Luke brought with him seemed to confirm the diagnosis of two herniated discs. However, the condition that had caused the herniation was not clear. Luke wasn't old enough for degeneration to have occurred, and there was no evidence of any kind of fracture or other trauma. The AK practitioner knew that she had to find the cause of the problem before she could treat it properly.

Gait analysis revealed that Luke walked in a hunched over manner, revealing a tightness of his hip flexors. Even though his pain was on the right, the doctor noticed that Luke slightly dragged his left leg behind him. Postural Analysis also revealed that Luke was barely able to straighten up fully due to the pain and leaned slightly to the left. His range of motion was severely diminished, and his right leg was so weak he was unable to toe walk or heel walk.

They moved to the examination room. Due to Postural and Gait Analysis, the doctor suspected a problem with Luke's left psoas muscle. The psoas muscles are important low back muscles on either side of the lumbar spine and attach to the discs between the vertebrae. Any dysfunction in these muscles can lead to a disc bulge or herniation. The doctor asked him to lie face up on the table.

Surprised, Luke said that he had never lied face up on a chiropractic table because the previous doctor only had him go face down to examine his spine. The Applied Kinesiologist related to him that very often back symptoms stem from a problem in the front of the body and a key to helping severe low back pain comes from treating important core muscles such as the abdominals and psoas.

The doctor tested these muscles and found no weakness at first. Then she retested the muscle immediately after the first test. This time the left psoas muscle tested as severely inhibited. Luke groaned in pain. This weakness pattern confirmed the need for the AK technique known as Strain Counter Strain Trigger Point Release. Unlike the more commonly known Travell trigger point condition in which shortening of the fascial covering causes pain, a strain counter strain trigger point results in a dysfunction of the muscle due to the receptors or spindle cells located in the muscle itself.

The doctor explained that there was a problem in the muscles in his low back, but she could only get to the muscle from the front to treat it. She further explained that chronic inhibition of his left psoas muscle could lead to tightening of his right hip flexor muscle and was a critical, and usually overlooked, contributing factor to his low back pain on the right. She told him to relax as best he could while she palpated his abdominal region to test for any soreness. The doctor proceeded to position his thigh up close to his chest until she found a position that was the least painful for Luke. This position signaled the most likely point at which the psoas muscle was strained. She placed a Vibracussor®, a deep percussion device, over the center of the psoas muscle and held the position for 90 seconds. The doctor let the leg down and retested the muscle. It was strong, and Luke's pain had lessened. This technique effectively "resets" the spindle cell receptors so that they are able to send the proper signals to the muscle, and it can resume its normal function of stabilizing the low back.

Now that Luke was a little more comfortable, the doctor had him turn over and lie face down. She examined his low back region by pushing on individual vertebra to see if they were moving freely and independently. She found that they were not. The doctor diagnosed that Luke was suffering from several lumbar spinal fixations.

Spinal fixation is a condition in which several of the vertebrae become immobilized or "locked together" as a unit instead of moving flexibly. This "locking up" of the spine occurs due to a forced restriction of natural movements and can lead to herniated or swollen discs and, if not treated, to some level of permanent disc degeneration.

The most common causes of this forced restriction of natural movement include walking with your hands in your pockets, carrying a heavy backpack or handbag, or even holding a phone in one position for long periods. In other words, any activity that does not allow for the free movement of the arms that provide a complimentary counter-rotation of the spine to balance those occurring with the free movement of the legs will result in these spinal fixations. The tension caused by this unnatural restriction causes tautness in the deep intrinsic muscles of the spine. Over time, this tension leads to spasms of these muscles that connect directly to the vertebrae and eventually leads to a restriction of movement or a "locking up." In turn, these spinal fixations perpetuate the hypertonicity (spasm) of the muscles. It's a vicious cycle that can then lead to muscle inhibition patterns, disc problems, stenosis, spinal degeneration and eventually severe pain. Spinal fixations in younger patients, usually from book-laden backpacks, can lead to scoliosis. It can only be corrected by precise spinal manipulation of the affected spinal segments.

Luke's case is typical in that the spinal restrictions are not initially painful and are easily ignored. Gradually, the condition worsens to where it builds up to the point that the pain is brutal, and the patient believes he "just woke up with it." Luke had been creating this condition for years, unwittingly, by walking asymmetrically with one arm restricted while carrying his heavy sample case or from long conversations on his phone.

Using a specialized adjusting tool named an Arthrostim®, the doctor was able to release the spinal fixations by applying a gentle impulse on two adjacent vertebrae in opposite directions and restore the normal free movement to each individual bone in the lumbar spine. This counter-rotation correction frees the individual vertebra from each other and releases the perpetual muscle spasm that has been keeping the vertebrae locked in place.

Once the vertebrae were moving freely, the doctor performed the Disc Pump Technique to relieve pressure and separate the vertebrae from each other. The doctor used her hands to perform this therapy for 15 repetitions. Afterward, ice packs were placed over the area for 20 minutes to help relieve any swelling.

After the ice packs were removed, Luke gingerly got off the table. He could stand much straighter and was able to walk almost normally. His pain had diminished substantially as well. He hesitated before sitting down to put on his shoes on but was relieved when he was able to do so without severe pain.

He was told to ice his low back for 20 minutes every hour, for a maximum of 6 times per day, until his next appointment the following week. Luke was given a list of natural supplements including vitamin C and manganese to help heal the disc, along with omega 3 oils, boswellia, and curcumin to relieve inflammation and pain. The doctor encouraged him to limit sitting; and when he did sit, to avoid leaning forward during the treatment period. This is critically important because sitting, and especially leaning forward, increases the intradiscal pressure—possibly resulting in a relapse.

The examination during the next visit revealed that Luke was much improved. His pain had reached a more manageable level, and his gait and posture were close to normal. The doctor performed pulse-point analysis of the acupuncture meridian system. Acupuncture has been proven highly effective in cases of low back pain. The analysis revealed an imbalance in the bladder meridian that runs down the entire spine and the back of the legs. The doctor used a retractable acupuncture device (a Tei-Shin) to treat the imbalance. Luke experienced more mobility than he had before the acupuncture treatment and felt a dramatic decrease in his pain level.

Luke required two treatments a week for two months and then one per week for four months due to the extent of his disc herniations. Even before his full treatment was complete, he was back to working full days, driving to his appointments, and enjoying his regular activities. He replaced his heavy sample case with one with wheels and alternated the use of his arms when pulling it, as well as using a hands-free device during his follow-up phone calls to avoid impeding free arm movement when walking. Completely healed, Luke has experienced no back or leg pain and has resumed his very active lifestyle.

* * *

Your low back is critically important to your overall mobility and strength. When the low back is compromised, it can render sitting, standing, walking, and even lying down a living hell. No matter how strong you may be, when you are suffering from low back pain, it saps the life out of you.

Proponents of traditional medicine maintain a nearly knee-jerk reaction to low back pain that begins with various medications such as NSAIDs and opioids, ultimately progressing through steroid injections, and ending with some kind of surgery. However, NSAIDs have serious side effects, opioids can be highly addictive, steroid injections provide only temporary relief, and spinal surgery doesn't always relieve the symptoms or underlying condition. Additionally, the risks of permanent nerve damage with back surgery are high as well. Progressive medical experts prefer the non-pharmaceutical approach and understand the critical importance of addressing the physical components of low back pain.

The AK and integrative medicine approach to low back conditions can relieve and/or cure low back pain and promote ongoing health in people suffering from nonpathological cases by isolating the fundamental causes and treating them. Spinal adjustments, muscle manipulation techniques, acupuncture therapies, cranial-sacral corrections, exercise, stress reduction, and good nutrition all play a vital role in relieving low back pain and keeping your lower back in prime condition.

9

SPORTS INJURIES AND TRAUMA

Sports and sports-related activities put an enormous strain on the body. Athletes, both professional and amateur, need to be able to respond on command with speed, strength, precision, dexterity, and endurance while being able to employ superior decision making under pressure. They tend to push their bodies to the limit, which increases the chances of injury. However, many sports-related injuries can be prevented by maintaining the individual's systems at a high level of function through proper muscular-bone alignments and optimal nutritional support. When accidents happen, a well-functioning body can heal more quickly.

Sports injuries are generally the result of either repetitive motion or trauma. Serious strength training with weights can lead to shoulder problems; running often causes shin splints or runner's knee; basketball players are prone to Achilles tendonitis; tennis players often develop elbow, wrist and shoulder problems—all due to the repetitive motions required by these sports. Traumatic injuries are usually caused by singular events such as falling, colliding with other players, and engaging in extreme movements that damage muscles, bones, and joints.

Mechanically speaking, sports injuries are not much different from other physical injuries. Whether it's running up a flight of steps, carrying a heavy bag, or lifting a toddler the wrong way, any unusual movement can compromise muscles or cause misalignment of bones. In sports, the movements are often more intense and frequent, but the effects on the body are similar. In either case, the key to recovery is proper diagnosis of the specific injury as early as possible, as well as taking the appropriate measures to treat it so that the body will heal itself.

When a person is accustomed to a routine of regular exercise or sports activity, his or her body adapts to the physiological and emotional benefits of it. You feel healthier, look better, and have a sense of accomplishment at achieving your personal best. Competitive or professional athletes have additional concerns about maintaining careers, college scholarships, and the general prestige that comes from being a winner. However, an injury that prevents him or her from engaging in a preferred activity not only disrupts physiological well-being, but also increases the psychological pressure to heal and get "back in the game" as quickly as possible. This pressure can often prove to be a challenge to an individual's health and forces many to resume their activity before their bodies are ready. Many people take what they think are shortcuts offered by traditional medicine, such as medication to mask the pain or unnecessary surgery that promises to "fix" the problem. These treatments are often not effective and can actually have adverse long-term effects.

Another concern regarding the treatment of sports injuries is premature physical therapy (PT). The goal of PT is to help injured muscles and tendons strengthen and heal. It is vitally important for the recovery from all sports-related injuries. However, PT is most effective when the muscles and tendons are strong enough to accept it. If the body is out of alignment, or if the muscles and tendons are physiologically inhibited, this important rehabilitation does not have the desired result, and the recovery period will be longer. One of the singular benefits of AK is that it physiologically prepares the body for the healing process of PT. As stated earlier, *physiological therapy* (AK) should always precede *physical therapy* (PT).

Applied Kinesiology helps in the prevention of, and effective recovery from, sports injuries by keeping your body's biomechanical systems balanced and functioning properly without invasive medical procedures.

SELECTED INJURIES RELATED TO SPORTS ACTIVITY

CONCUSSIVE HEAD INJURY

Your brain is the most complex organ in your body, containing over 100 billion nerve cells and trillions of nerve pathways. It weighs 3 pounds and uses approximately 25% of your body's total oxygen. The brain is a delicate structure that has the same consistency as gelatin and is protected by the bones of the skull, three thin membranes known as meninges, and the cerebrospinal fluid-which acts as a shock absorber to cushion the brain inside your skull. A violent blow directly to any part of the head or a sudden acceleration/deceleration of the head (such as a car accident or bodily collision with another person) can cause your brain to be pushed hard against the inner walls of your skull, causing some level of traumatic brain injury (TBI) or concussion. Concussions can affect brain function due to damage to the brain cells and inflammation from the collision of the brain with the inside of the skull.

The symptoms of a concussion may include the following: headaches, ear ringing, dizziness, floating visual images, double vision, nausea or vomiting, slurred speech, confusion, balance problems, temporary loss of consciousness and loss of memory (usually about the traumatic event itself). Many symptoms are often delayed for hours or days after the incident such as changes in taste or smell; problems with concentration and memory; sensitivity to light and noise; sleep disturbances; seizures; and personality changes including irritability and depression. This delayed reaction is known as Post-Concussion Syndrome.

While concussions can happen to anyone at any time, they occur most frequently during sports activities. An estimated 1.6–3.8 million sports and recreation-related concussions occur yearly in the United States.[21] The National Safety Council states that 10% of contact athletes will suffer a concussion yearly.[22] Sports concussions are rising, with an estimated 15% of all high school students experiencing 1 or more concussions in 2017, with 6% reporting two or more.[23] High school football accounts for 47% of all reported sports concussions,[24] followed by hockey and soccer.

Statistics reveal that while one concussion can be problematic, it is the subsequent head traumas that are the cause of permanent brain damage. Cumulative sports concussions have shown to increase the likelihood of permanent neurological disability by 39%.[24] Since 90% of concussions do NOT involve loss of consciousness,[25] it is critical to know that the signs and symptoms of a concussion are often subtle in nature. Until proven otherwise, doctors, athletes, parents, and coaches should treat any head injury as a traumatic brain injury (TBI) and take all necessary precautions to properly test and then treat it appropriately.

One of the most serious conditions associated with head concussions is Chronic Traumatic Encephalopathy (CTE). This is a progressive degenerative disease that affects the brains of people who have suffered repeated concussions or other head injuries. CTE is a serious pathological disease, formerly called *dementia pugillistica,* that was predominately found in boxers due to the repetitive blows to the head that they suffered. It has now been diagnosed in football players and represents a pathological condition that has progressed beyond the scope of functional medicine, including AK, to treat or cure.

There are three levels of concussion: Grade 1 is considered mild, with symptoms such as dizziness lasting under fifteen minutes and no loss of consciousness; Grade 2 is considered moderate, with symptoms such as dizziness, nausea or disorientation lasting over fifteen minutes and no loss of consciousness; Grade 3 is considered severe, with loss of consciousness and sustained serious physiological and mental symptoms.

Diagnosing concussions is complicated and expensive. There is no single test to diagnose a concussion definitively. Most patients suspected of suffering a concussion undergo a neurological examination and, depending upon the findings, may have a CT scan and/or an MRI. Unfortunately, these tests are not entirely conclusive. Since many patients don't exhibit any serious symptoms after the injury, they often don't get the appropriate tests until the condition has progressed too far. However, a new blood test named the Brain

Trauma Indicator, approved by the Food and Drug Administration in February 2018,[26] and an Eye Tracking Test, approved in January 2019,[27] may allow doctors to diagnose a concussion soon after the incident occurs.

The generally accepted measure for diagnosing concussions is the Glasgow Coma Scale. After a series of physical tests regarding eyesight, verbal and motor responses, a specialist can arrive at a cumulative score on this scale. In conjunction with head scans and blood tests, the doctor is then able to reliably ascertain whether a patient has had a concussion and the possible extent of damage it has caused. Doctors have become more proactive in using these diagnostic techniques soon after a head injury has occurred.

* * *

BETH, 17, was an accomplished high school soccer player. During a game, she was jumping to head the ball when her head violently collided with the shoulder of another player. Stunned by the collision, Beth was taken out of the game due to fear of a concussion. While she displayed no serious symptoms, the coach kept her out of the game to avoid the possibility of Second Impact Syndrome. Second Impact Syndrome is a condition that occurs when a second trauma to the head occurs before the brain has fully recovered from the first concussion. This syndrome causes rapid and severe brain swelling and can have catastrophic results, including death.

Her parents took her to a nearby emergency room and explained what had happened. The doctor conducted a neurological assessment. Although the tests did not reveal any immediate danger, he reported that, given the power of the collision, she might have suffered a Grade 1 concussion. Beth's mother, who was an emergency room nurse at that hospital, was a bit skeptical of the diagnosis. She had seen patients come into the ER with concussions, and Beth didn't display any of the usual symptoms.

Two days later, Beth started to have headaches, so her parents brought her for a CT scan. Concussions do not show up on CT scans, but brain swelling (edema), bruising, and bleeding do. The CT scan results came back normal; thereby, ruling out a life-threatening brain injury. Her doctor suggested that Beth take some over-the-counter pain medication to help with the painful headaches.

Another week went by, and Beth still had headaches along with ringing in her ears and neck pains. The ER doctor's suggestion that she could have suffered a Grade 1 concussion seemed to be correct. Beth went back to her medical doctor, who said that sometimes these symptoms are associated with Post-Concussion Syndrome and could last for a few months. He referred Beth to a neurologist, who ordered an MRI. The results also came back negative for any pathology, which meant Beth might be suffering the routine after-effects of a minor concussion.

Beth's symptoms persisted. She couldn't concentrate at school or resume playing soccer. Beth's mom decided to get a second opinion from the Applied Kinesiologist who had treated her in the past for various sports-related injuries.

During the consultation, Beth described what had happened at the game. Her headaches, dizziness, and ringing in her ears had started to develop a few days after the injury—they were driving her crazy. She was concerned that she'd miss the entire soccer season if she waited until they subsided.

The doctor examined the test results from her visit to the hospital and the neurologist. All the tests were negative for severe traumatic brain injury (TBI) but did not conclusively rule out a Grade 1 concussion. He saw that her pupils were of equal sizes and constricted normally when a light was flashed in her eyes. She was able to move her eyes smoothly in all directions and was able to focus her gaze on the ceiling and on the doctor's finger when he brought it to her nose. She was able to smile, stick out her tongue without deviation, and had normal gag reflexes. As her responses were all normal, it seemed that it was unlikely that she had suffered a Grade 1 concussion. Something else was causing her symptoms.

Postural Analysis revealed her head (occiput) to be elevated and rotated slightly to the left. Gait Analysis displayed some unsteadiness and the same elevation of the occiput on her left as well. He examined her head and neck. Beth had limited ability to turn her head to the right. She was also unable to bend her head and neck to the left toward her shoulder. Both of these particular restrictions indicated an issue with her neck and head muscles, specifically the sternocleidomastoid and upper trapezius muscles, whose function is to help turn the head to the right and bend it to the left. Both of these muscles are partially controlled by a cranial nerve called the spinal accessory nerve, which exits through a small opening called the jugular foramen. This opening is formed by the union of the occipital and temporal bones.

Through a combination of Therapy Localization (placing the patient's hand over specific points on the body); Respiratory Challenging (having the patient hold certain breathing patterns); Structural Challenging (in this case, inducing specific motion into different bones of the skull); and Functional Muscle Testing (FMT), the doctor found that these two neck muscles initially showed weakness (physiological inhibition) and then regained strength (physiological facilitation) during restricted respiration. This led the doctor to believe that the cranial nerve that controls these muscles was somehow compromised.

Next, the Applied Kinesiologist examined Beth's skull bones. The skull is comprised of twenty-two bones and approximately eighty-six joints. The diameter of the skull expands and contracts 2.2mm every ten seconds in distinct patterns. Any lack of movement of your skull bones can affect general brain function and, more specifically, the twelve cranial nerves that are housed within your cranium. These twelve nerves, which can be thought of as *modified spinal nerves*, control a wide variety of sensory and bodily functions including smell, eyesight, hearing, taste, facial sensation and expression, neck movement, speech, swallowing, balance, digestion, heart rate, and blood pressure—as well as general relaxation. They are highly susceptible to a variety of physiological factors, chief among them being head injury.

The doctor diagnosed that the source of her symptoms was the restriction of the *spinal accessory nerve* and, in all likelihood, the *acoustic nerve*. This would explain the ear ringing and her dizziness since the acoustic (vestibulocochlear) nerve controls balance and orientation along with hearing. Beth's symptoms could be due to the compression of the bones that form the jugular foramen opening and the internal acoustic meatus (inner ear canal) where these two cranial nerves, respectively, pass through. In other words, Beth's condition was caused by a dysfunction of the cranial bones from the trauma of the initial collision on the field and was probably never a concussion.

Beth and her parents were relieved at the doctor's diagnosis. It seemed to make sense to them, as all the clinical and sensory tests did not indicate that she had suffered a concussion, but it was obvious something was not right. They asked: what can be done? The doctor related that once pathologies such as skull fractures or internal bleeding are ruled out, AK can help people with head injuries, including concussions, by using functional modalities to restore the skull's inherent flexibility and subsequently relieve pressure on the brain and the cranial nerves.

Treatment consisted of the doctor gently applying pressure to the temporal bones on the left side of her head for several repetitions as Beth breathed deeply. After these light skull manipulations, the doctor placed ice packs wrapped in cloth around Beth's head for twenty minutes. He recommended that she do this for twenty minutes every hour, for a maximum of eight times daily, when at home for the next three days.

When the doctor brought Beth up and off the table, she said that she felt much better. Her headache and ringing in her ears were nearly gone. The doctor tested the two neck muscles and noted that they were now functioning normally. Beth moved her head more freely. He recommended that she take fish oil capsules, blueberry extract, and the herb turmeric to help with any inflammation from the compression; as well as a B-vitamin complex that contained activated B6, folic acid and B12, along with choline and inositol—all of which are crucial to brain function. He told her to increase her water intake to sixty-four ounces daily and to be sure to hydrate regularly. She was instructed to engage in twenty to thirty minutes of brisk walking daily (as long as symptoms did not worsen) since light aerobic activity can help speed recovery of concussions and head injuries in general.

Beth required four more treatments, after which she was back to playing soccer—but was a bit more vigilant on the field.

TENNIS ELBOW

The elbow is a complex hinge joint formed between the upper arm and the forearm. The bone in the upper arm is called the humerus, while the two bones in the forearm are known as the ulna and the radius. It is comprised of three separate joints: the humeroulnar, the humeroradial, and the proximal radioulnar. The first two are traditionally thought of as the elbow *per se*. The elbow flexes (bends) and straightens (extends) at these first two joints. The pivoting function of the radioulnar allows for the rotation of the elbow. This motion is known as supination/pronation.

The main muscles of the elbow are the biceps, triceps, supinator, and pronator teres. The biceps and triceps are most important in the flexing and straightening of your elbow joint. The supinator, with help from the biceps, rotates your forearm at the elbow so your palm is facing upward. The pronator teres rotates the forearm at the elbow so your palm is facing downward.

These muscular connections and movements give the elbow a profound and deep relationship with the shoulder and wrist. The biceps and triceps not only bend and straighten the elbow; they also flex and extend the arm at the shoulder. Supination and pronation involve the entire forearm all the way down to your wrist. In fact, due to the biceps function in supination (turning the palm upward) and the fact that there is another pronator muscle at the radioulnar joint down by the wrist (pronator quadratus), explains why when your elbow is compromised—it can directly affect the functioning of the shoulder and wrist as well.

The ulnar collateral ligament (UCL) is a ligament on the inner side of your elbow that helps to stabilize the elbow joint by connecting the upper arm (humerus) to one of the forearm bones (ulna). Because this ligament is such an important stabilizer of the inner elbow, sports medicine orthopedic specialists have developed a specific test to evaluate its function known as the Valgus Stress Test. Many agree that this test is more effective than an X-ray or MRI in determining the integrity of this important ligament. It is a simple test, whereby the doctor applies pressure to the outside of the elbow while holding the forearm of the patient and administers a slight inwards (Valgus) pressure. If the patient experiences pain or if the doctor notices excessive movement, a problem with the UCL is indicated—possibly a strain or tear. Applied Kinesiologists also use this maneuver to uncover a misalignment (subluxation) of the elbow. This bony misalignment creates an intense strain to the UCL and may be the leading predisposing factor for rupture of the ligament.

A tear of the UCL and the loud popping sound that accompanies it occurs as a result of the strain from a series of repetitive motions that precede the actual traumatic event. Applied Kinesiology procedures can prove extremely beneficial in helping an athlete recover from a serious sprain or partial tear. More importantly, it helps to prevent this condition in the first place by ensuring that the elbow, forearm and shoulder muscles are functioning properly and that all corresponding bones are in proper alignment. A Major League Baseball trainer expressed it succinctly: "If you have a posture problem, you have an elbow problem, and you have a shoulder problem." It is also important that the leg and core (abdominals, back and pelvic) muscles are functioning optimally to ensure proper biomechanics in the overhand motion that usually causes injuries to the UCL.

One of the most common and painful conditions that affect the elbow is lateral epicondylitis, also known as *tennis elbow*. Tennis elbow is technically caused by microtears in the tendons of muscles, usually of the wrist extensor muscles, on the outer part of the elbow (lateral epicondyle). The wrist flexor and extensor muscles connect to the inner and outer sides of the elbow, respectively. After hundreds of repetitive motions that strain and tear the same tendon(s) each time, a single traumatic event can disable the entire arm—causing excruciating pain. If the damage is a serious tear in the tendon, it probably will require surgery, physical therapy, and a long recovery period. If the pain is due to the culmination of microtears exacerbated by one particularly strong movement, without a serious tear, AK will help restore full function to the muscle, tendon, and joint without any invasive procedures.

* * *

FERNANDO, 28, was a prominent tennis instructor at a prestigious tennis club. During a practice session, he hit a backhand shot hard and felt a sharp pain in the outer part of his right elbow. Over the years, he had experienced variants of this kind of pain; he would just play through it, grab the acetaminophen in his locker between clients, wait for the pain to subside, and then continue playing. However, this time, instead of subsiding, the pain intensified to the point that he had to cancel the rest of his clients for the day. He went home, applied ice and took painkillers. Unfortunately, the pain did not get any better.

He had never experienced this level of pain before. The pain got so bad that he had to cancel his upcoming sessions until he could find relief. He made an appointment with the orthopedist affiliated with the club. He examined his elbow and took some X-rays. The X-rays essentially ruled out any pathological conditions, such as fractures or tumors. Based upon Fernando's symptoms and physical examination, the orthopedist diagnosed his patient's condition as tennis elbow (lateral epicondylitis). He suggested that Fernando keep up with the ice, rest, and switch to ibuprofen, instead of acetaminophen, to help with the pain and inflammation.

After a week of no improvement, the doctor decided to give Fernando a cortisone shot. Cortisone is a prescription drug usually coupled with some kind pain suppressant injected into a joint to relieve inflammation and pain. If taken too frequently, it can cause deterioration and permanent damage. The shot helped, but after a few days, the pain returned.

The orthopedic specialist suggested more aggressive procedures since none of these treatments were working. One method involved a dry needling procedure, wherein a needle pierces the damaged tendon in several places in the hopes of inducing a healing response. Another is ultrasonic tenotomy (TENEX), wherein a needle is inserted into your elbow, and ultrasonic waves liquefy the damaged tissue (usually tendon and muscle) which is then sucked out. If neither of these very painful treatment methods is successful, the final solution involves surgery—where one large or several small incisions are made to remove the damaged tissue. All of these expensive treatments require a long recovery period and physical therapy.

Fernando was concerned. Not only could he not afford any of these complex medical treatments, but he also could not afford to lose weeks, perhaps months, of time away from the court and his clients. He had known colleagues who had undergone surgery, and they never played quite as well as they did before or had to give up tennis entirely.

Fortunately, one of his older colleagues who had experienced a variety of conditions including tennis elbow over the years had a suggestion for him. He said he had undergone the full range of non-surgical medical treatments, but that he had received the most relief from a specialist who employed an alternative therapy called AK. Fernando was desperate for relief, so he took the doctor's information and made an appointment for an evaluation.

During the consultation, Fernando shared his medical reports with the doctor. He was concerned that his orthopedist was unable to help him either with painkillers or cortisone. "Taking medications to block pain signals is like disengaging the smoke detector in your house," the doctor said. "Without adequate warning, the fire could become serious. Pain is the body's warning signal that something is wrong. We need to pay attention to it, not mask it, because the condition could get worse the longer we allow it to go on."

He also mentioned that his orthopedist had suggested several invasive procedures that he was only interested in pursuing if it were the last resort. The AK doctor assured him that she would do everything in her power to get him playing tennis again, without having to undergo these treatments.

The doctor noticed that he wore a soft neoprene elbow compression sleeve. "Does the sleeve help to relieve any of your pain?" she asked.

"A little," Fernando replied. He said that he routinely wore it on the court in the hopes of preventing a problem like this and was wearing it when he got injured.

The doctor began her examination by asking Fernando to remove the soft elbow brace and then proceeded to have the patient stand and then walk. Postural and Gait Analysis showed that his right hand and wrist were slightly flexed inwards and rotated with the palm tensely facing his side as if he were going to draw a gun from his holster during a gunfight in a western movie.

The AK practitioner proceeded to palpate the outer part of the elbow (lateral epicondyle). Fernando winced in pain. The doctor then placed a Dynamometer, a standard medical device that measures hand strength, in Fernando's right hand and had him squeeze it, then again in his left hand. His right-hand grip test caused pain in his elbow and registered 50% weaker than his left hand, even though he was right-handed.

The doctor then performed Kaplan's Test. Kaplan's Test involves having the patient squeeze the Dynamometer to get a baseline strength measure. The doctor then repeats the test, this time squeezing together the elbow joint (the proximal radioulnar joint). If the grip is stronger than the first measurement, it indicates that the patient is suffering from tennis elbow. Fernando tested positive for this condition and also noted that his pain lessened when the doctor squeezed the joint.

The doctor instructed Fernando to put the soft brace back on and again performed Kaplan's Test. The weakness and pain were the same as at the initial testing. Generally, compression sleeves add some support, but they also lessen the ability of the muscle to pull; thereby, reducing performance and altering joint dynamics. This can lead to further injury and pain under the strain of sports activity. The doctor replaced the compression sleeve with a Gel Arc Elbow Brace which is designed specifically for this condition. It maintains the elbow joint in alignment and, with its dual-sided gel arc, reduces the muscle tension at the outer part of the elbow (lateral epicondyle). She had Fernando perform the test again. This time Fernando's grip was stronger and much less painful.

The doctor employed AK muscle testing, which revealed a weakness of the wrist extensor muscles (extensor carpi ulnaris and extensor carpi radialis). Next, using Therapy Localization, she had Fernando place his hand over the lateral epicondyle where the wrist extensors muscles connect. Fernando shared that he felt the pain in the same exact point in the elbow after his backhand shot. The doctor again tested the muscles; the pain was diminished, and the muscles now tested stronger. Additional testing revealed a fascial shortening of the supinator muscle that connects to the lateral epicondyle, resulting in weakness. The supinator muscle plays a key role in backhand tennis swings.

After ascertaining the various impaired muscle components of Fernando's problem, the doctor proceeded to perform the Extremity Challenge to the elbow joint for misalignments. The doctor found that the radial head, the bone that connects to the lateral epicondyle of the upper arm bone (humerus), had become improperly aligned. The doctor palpated the area, and it was acutely painful.

The doctor had Fernando taste, not swallow, a natural "antihistamine" supplement that contained vitamin C, perilla extract and quercetin. After Fernando noted that he could taste it by confirming its slight acidity, the doctor tested the wrist extensor muscles, and they now tested stronger. Fernando stated that the pain was greatly diminished and was amazed that a simple taste of this supplement could relieve the pain better than synthetic drugs.

The doctor explained this AK technique. When there is damage to the mast cells located in connective tissue such as a joint capsule, tendon, or ligament, and there is localized inflammation—natural substances that signal a pain response in the brain are released. These substances are called histamines. Stimulating the gustatory receptors in the tongue that carry the sensation of taste with a natural supplement that has "antihistamine" properties causes enough of a neurological impulse to create an immediate decrease in pain and improvement in muscle function.

The doctor explained to an astonished Fernando that, "the mechanism for this pain reduction while tasting specific nutrients has to do with the taste receptors on the tongue and their immediate influence on the autonomic nervous system which modulates pain sensation. Just like the autonomic response of sweating immediately after tasting a spicy chile pepper." Fernando nodded that he understood. The Applied Kinesiologist continued, "Likewise, when you taste something, it can improve physiological muscle function and performance due to the stimulation of nerves going from your tongue to the hypothalamus gland to the spinal cord to your muscles."

The doctor diagnosed Fernando with tennis elbow caused by an inhibition of muscles and misalignment of bones in the elbow-arm-wrist complex. The treatment began with the Origin/Insertion Technique to the strained wrist extensor muscles to help heal the microtears and facilitate the Golgi tendons to help strengthen (physiologically facilitate) the muscle and restore its normal function. Next, the doctor did a medical massage to release the tightened supinator muscle from its fascial shortening. She then adjusted the radial head to realign the elbow joint properly.

Fernando felt substantial relief from the pain. The doctor sent him away with the natural antihistamine supplement he had just tasted and instructed him to ingest one every two hours for the next three days. She also gave him the Gel Arc Elbow Brace to wear at all times until the next visit. Fernando was instructed to ice the elbow for twenty minutes every hour, up to twelve times a day, for the next week and refrain from playing tennis.

After his second treatment four days later, his condition was so improved that he could return to playing, so long as he avoided using the backhand shot. After the fourth treatment the following week, his condition was in complete remission, and he could play with no restrictions. To prevent this condition from recurring, the doctor instructed him on using a rubber band exercise to strengthen the forearm muscles and tendons, along with elbow rotational (supination/pronation) warm-up exercises before playing. He remains free of any residual pain, feels as strong as ever, and is back on the court.

WHIPLASH

Cervical whiplash syndrome, also known as hyperflexion-hyperextension injury, is a common traumatic injury to the muscles, ligaments and other structures of the cervical spine. A whiplash represents a neck sprain/strain that occurs from a jarring collision that causes a rapid back-and-forth movement of the neck, similar to the cracking of a whip. This injury is usually associated with an automobile accident, but whiplashes commonly result from sports accidents.

Approximately 1,000,000 people incur a whiplash injury yearly in the US with 25-40% of these cases resulting in chronic pain and disability.[28] Symptoms of a whiplash includes the following: neck pain and stiffness, headaches, pain between the shoulder blades or in the shoulder itself, dizziness, difficulty sleeping, trouble concentrating, and anxiety. Whiplash injuries rarely show up on X-rays, CT scans or MRIs since the pain and disability is primarily the result of soft tissue injuries.

Treatments generally consist of medications such as anti-inflammatories and muscle relaxers, followed by PT. These may temporarily relieve the pain and stiffness; but without addressing the injured muscles and misaligned spinal bones that accompany a whiplash injury, the benefits are generally not permanent and maximum function is rarely restored. Applied Kinesiologists are well trained to successfully treat people suffering from whiplash injuries and their treatments lead to a complete recovery.

* * *

DANIEL, 40, was a high-ranking city building official and an ex-collegiate basketball player. On weekends, he enjoyed playing pick-up games at his neighborhood basketball court to de-stress from his intense work schedule. During one game as he was passing the ball to a teammate, a player from the other team bulldozed into his left side. Daniel was hit so hard that he felt his neck whip back and forth quickly. He shook off the slight dizziness he felt and continued playing.

The next morning, Daniel woke up with excruciating neck pain. He could not move his head to the left at all or look down. He took a hot shower and some ibuprofen, but the pain continued. It was a weekend, and his regular doctor was not available; so he went to the local walk-in clinic where X-rays were taken. There were no fractures or dislocations, but there was a slight straightening and tilt of the cervical spine. After hearing about what happened at the game, the attending physician diagnosed it as cervical whiplash—caused by a sudden rapid back and forth movement of the head and neck. He prescribed ibuprofen and muscle relaxers (cyclobenzaprine). As there was no damage to the cervical spine, he said that the pain should subside in a few days. However, if it didn't, he suggested that he see his regular doctor.

Daniel found that the muscle relaxers simply made him drowsy, and the ibuprofen only upset his stomach and didn't help to dampen the pain. He went to see his general practitioner, who confirmed the diagnosis of whiplash. Daniel asked his doctor if he should wear a foam collar. The doctor said that studies have shown that collars often cause more harm than good and interfere with the natural healing process. The doctor asked if he wanted him to prescribe some stronger painkillers. Daniel passed on the drugs and accepted a prescription for physical therapy. But after one session, he was in such pain that he could not endure it and stopped going.

After three weeks of living with severe neck pain that was only relieved temporarily by a long hot shower, he was a physical wreck. He couldn't get comfortable at night due to the pain and wasn't getting enough sleep. Driving was dangerous, as he couldn't turn his head. At his wit's end, he began to reconsider taking prescription painkillers.

During a routine supervision of the inspection of a new local sports arena, the building inspector noticed that Daniel had a difficult time turning his head to the left. Daniel, who had known the man for years, shared his story about his whiplash injury. The inspector mentioned that he had a whiplash pain similar to Daniel's from a car accident. He had tried strong painkillers but couldn't tolerate their side effects. He also went through physical therapy and massage therapy, but nothing helped. His doctor suggested that he visit a chiropractor. He found one who was also certified in a specialization known as AK. The doctor worked to relax his muscles by improving muscular function first, then gently realigned his neck with precise adjustments. After a few treatments, he was completely cured.

Daniel immediately made an appointment with the AK specialist. At the first visit, he had difficulty filling out the new patient forms because looking down created stabbing pain in the back of his neck.

During the consultation, the doctor listened to Daniel's basketball story. He asked him if he was experiencing any numbness or tingling down his hands. He replied no. After reading the reports from the walk-in clinic and Daniel's doctor and the unsuccessful physical therapy, the doctor proceeded with the exam. Gait analysis revealed that his head was elevated and rotated slightly to the right; he was so unsteady that he scraped the wall several times with his right shoulder as he walked down the hall.

Postural Analysis confirmed his head to be slightly higher and rotated to the right. Range of motion studies revealed that Daniel could not turn his head to the left or look down without feeling a piercing pain in the back of his head and neck. The AK practitioner conducted orthopedic and neurological tests and found no indication of disc herniation or neurological deficit. Daniel had normal sensations and strength in his arms and hands.

The doctor then palpated the right sternocleidomastoid muscle (SCM), the main muscle in the front of the neck that turns the head to the left. The muscle originates from the top of the sternum (breastbone) and the clavicle (collarbone) and runs upward to insert in the mastoid part of the temporal bone in the skull. AK manual muscle testing uncovered a distinct weakness (physiological inhibition) in this muscle. Daniel replied that he did not notice pain there except when the doctor palpated it, and that he mostly felt the intense pain in the back of his neck. The doctor explained that when a muscle on one side is strained, the complementary or opposing muscle usually responds by going into spasm. In Daniel's case, the tight, painful muscles in the back of his neck were predominately coming from a strain of the muscle in the front of his neck.

The Applied Kinesiologist noted nodules in this muscle where it connects to the bones via the tendons. Further investigation revealed a thickening of the fascial covering of the neck extensor muscles in the back of the neck as well. The doctor used Therapy Localization and Vertebral Challenging to find that the occiput (skull) and the second cervical vertebra were misaligned and were contributing to the condition.

The doctor proceeded to gently perform the Origin/Insertion Technique to Daniel's right SCM muscle. After 30 seconds of therapy to the Golgi tendon receptors located at the ends of the muscles, the doctor stopped and retested the muscle. It was much stronger (physiologically facilitated). The doctor asked Daniel to try to turn his head to the left. To Daniel's surprise, he could move it more easily. The doctor proceeded to perform percussion therapy using the Vibracussor® on the back of the neck, and then he performed two precise chiropractic adjustments to restore normal alignment of Daniel's skull and the second vertebra.

After these treatments, Daniel was able to move his head fully to the left and look down with minimal pain. Ice was applied to the area for twenty minutes. The doctor recommended a natural anti-inflammatory and antihistamine supplement containing omega 3 oils, turmeric, boswellia, and quercetin—along with calcium to help heal the muscle strain and magnesium to act as a natural muscle relaxer for the tight muscles.

Daniel required seven treatments in total. Once his neck muscles were strong enough, he went back to physical therapy for several sessions. Finally, fully recuperated from his whiplash injury, he resumed his weekend basketball games.

* * *

Whether competing professionally or recreationally, sports activities often push our bodies and minds to the limit of their capabilities. This kind of physiological and emotional stress, while exhilarating, increases the possibility of injury and damage to the body. Unless there is some kind of pathological problem, such as a broken bone or muscle tear, traditional medical treatments, such as surgery or prescription painkillers, are often not effective in restoring the body's biomechanical functions after a sports injury because they do not address the underlying cause of the problem and can cause complications. Many of these injuries can be treated and cured successfully through the special, non-invasive techniques of AK.

While you cannot prevent unexpected sporting accidents—this is why they are called *accidents*—you can help your body lessen their effects by keeping your muscles and joints as strong and supple as possible through good nutrition, adequate hydration, and proper bone/muscle alignment. AK's unique comprehensive approach to the musculoskeletal system enables your doctor to detect potential weaknesses before they become problems and helps you avoid or minimize the effect of an injury should it occur. When there is an issue, it can pinpoint the exact cause of the problem, and relieve or eliminate pain while restoring proper function without drugs or surgery.

10

GASTROINTESTINAL CONDITIONS

Your gastrointestinal (GI) system consists of eight parts. Five of these are in your GI tract and are often referred to as the "hollow digestive organs." They provide space for the passage of food and include the mouth, esophagus, stomach, small intestine, and large intestine. The other three fleshy or "solid organs" are the liver, gall bladder, and pancreas—all of which add secretions to help you digest, absorb, and eliminate everything you eat and drink.

Digestion is critically important because your bodily processes require energy from the nutrients contained in the foods and liquids you consume. The processes begin when the food enters your mouth. As you chew, food is broken down mechanically into small pieces. Saliva begins the chemical process of digestion, with the enzyme amylase, by breaking down starches like rice, pasta, and bread. After you swallow, the bolus or mashed up food enters the esophagus, where it is pushed down through the wave-like contractions (peristalsis) of the smooth muscle lining most of this muscular tube. This churned food lands in your stomach.

Your stomach is a muscular organ located on the upper left side of your abdomen just below your ribcage. Here, the gastric juices consisting of hydrochloric acid (HCl), sodium chloride and potassium chloride works to break down food to the molecular level.

The muscles in the stomach churn the food and then propel the digested food forward to the small intestine. Nutrients are then extracted and absorbed into the body. Waste moves to the large intestine and is eventually eliminated. The whole digestive process, from swallowing to absorption to elimination, takes approximately ten hours to three days, depending on various factors such as your digestive health and what you eat.

An often overlooked aspect of your digestive system is the complex relationship between the GI tract organs and their positioning within the body. Like other internal organs, the GI tract organs are held in place by various connective tissues and muscles, especially the abdominal and psoas muscles. Any dysfunction of these muscles can affect the digestive process. The overall system is mostly autonomous, kept in motion mainly by the parasympathetic nervous system and most notably by the vagus nerve, the longest of the cranial nerves. The vagus originates in the skull, travels down through an opening known as the jugular foramen, and supplies both sensory and motor functions to much of the digestive tract. Your vagus nerve is important for the proper healthy function of your GI tract and enhances the ability of the stomach to process food. This nerve is stimulated by, among other things, gentle exercise. This helps to explain why a leisurely walk after a meal helps with digestion.

Aside from serious pathological conditions, such as cancer, systemic chemical imbalances, and organ deformity, most GI conditions can be treated effectively by the unique biomechanical therapies of AK. Since so much of the proper function of these organs depends upon the health of the muscles, bones, and nerves that surround them, AK provides valuable assistance through the physical manipulation of muscles and organs, mechanical corrections to your cranium, chiropractic spinal adjustments, acupuncture therapies, and nutritional/herbal remedies. AK's physiologically-based therapies can help relieve the cause of the pain, bloating and discomfort in many people commonly diagnosed with GI conditions including stomach ulcers, acid reflux or GERD, inflammatory bowel disease (IBD), malabsorption syndrome, irritable bowel syndrome (IBS), and constipation.

ESOPHAGEAL/STOMACH PROBLEMS

Acid reflux or GERD (gastroesophageal reflux disease) is becoming a national epidemic with some statistics showing it afflicting up to 95,000,000 Americans yearly.[29] The symptoms include a burning sensation in your chest (heartburn), chest pain, lump in your throat, difficulty swallowing, bad breath, and regurgitation of food or liquid back into your throat or mouth. Most traditional treatments involve managing these symptoms through medications and dietary changes, neither of which address the various fundamental sources of the disorder.

In most instances, the underlying cause of GERD is a hiatal hernia. It occurs when the upper part of the stomach, which is connected to the lower esophageal sphincter (LES), slides up above the diaphragm. The LES is a muscular valve that closes as soon as food passes through it to prevent gastric acid from seeping upward in the esophagus and throat. Your diaphragm is a large dome-shaped muscle that separates your chest cavity from your abdominal cavity and regulates breathing. Normally, your stomach sits below the diaphragm. When it slides above the diaphragm, it can impact the function of the LES and cause acid to leak or "reflux" into the esophagus, causing the sensations of "heartburn" and burning in the throat.

While your stomach is designed to contain its powerful acid, your esophagus is not. Left untreated, the constant intrusion of acid into the esophagus can permanently affect its tissue and increase the risks of esophageal adenocarcinoma. People suffering from GERD find their quality of life severely affected. Their eating and sleeping habits become limited. Constant use of "heartburn" or "indigestion" medications can alter the digestive capabilities of the entire system and cause permanent damage as well.

* * *

GLORIA, 28, a high school science teacher, suffered from chronic, mild heartburn and slight burning pain in her throat. When it occurred, she would take some over the counter heartburn medications known as Histamine 2 blockers. (H2 blockers). These drugs include Nexium, Tagamet, Pepcid, or Zantac, and work by suppressing your stomach acid by blocking the histamine receptors in acid-producing cells in the stomach.

When she had a particularly severe bout of indigestion, she switched to a different class of over-the-counter drugs—proton pump inhibitors (PPIs). PPIs help with the symptoms of heartburn and acid reflux by reducing the amount of acid your stomach produces at the cellular level. Common PPIs such as Prilosec and Prevacid do this by blocking the enzyme in the wall of your stomach that produces the acid by shutting down the proton pumps that are necessary to create the energy to make acid. After a few days, the symptoms usually became more tolerable. Gloria excluded fatty, as well as spicy and acidic, foods from her diet and just managed the condition.

However, one day while attending a street fair she went off her diet by eating a sausage hero. In the days that followed, she had severe indigestion accompanied by acid reflux, chest pain, and difficulty swallowing. None of her usual remedies relieved her symptoms. Her discomfort grew so much that she went to her medical doctor, who diagnosed with her with GERD and prescribed a stronger PPI medication.

While the stronger medications helped mitigate the symptoms, Gloria was concerned that they could affect her overall health if she took them over a sustained period. She went back to her medical doctor and shared her concerns. The doctor referred her to a gastroenterologist. At first, the specialist suggested trying different medications, but Gloria resisted and wanted to understand what was causing the condition. The gastroenterologist had an X-ray taken that revealed that Gloria's stomach had slid up past her diaphragm, indicating a hiatal hernia. He then suggested a barium X-ray study to confirm the diagnosis. Reluctant to take this test due to the radiation, she agreed to take a sonogram instead. This ultrasound examination confirmed his diagnosis.

The doctor told Gloria that surgery was required to bring the stomach back down to its normal position to cure the problem. Not wanting to have surgery, Gloria asked her doctor about alternatives. The doctor then gave her a list of lifestyle changes such as sleeping at an elevated angle; avoiding heavy meals as well as tomatoes, onions, spicy food and soda; not lying down right after eating; and continued use of the medication. Gloria had been doing all of these things already, and, while they helped, she still suffered.

Gloria was at her wit's end. The burning sensation in her chest and throat was unbearable. She ate less and less due to the regurgitation of food and worsening heartburn. Another teacher at the school, concerned that Gloria was losing too much weight, asked if everything was okay. Gloria shared with her the situation. Her colleague commiserated; it turned out that her husband also suffered from a hiatal hernia. He had to sleep in a recliner to relieve the pain at night for years. "How is he now?" Gloria asked. "He's fine," replied her friend. Surprised, she asked, "Did he have surgery to correct it?" The woman shook her head. "We found a doctor who was able to cure him without it. He's an expert in alternative therapies." Gloria took the name and made an appointment.

Upon arriving at the office, she filled out the patient profile forms and was escorted to the consultation room. During the patient consultation, Gloria shared her sausage story and the worsening of symptoms, which included shortness of breath. She brought along her X-ray and sonogram results as well. After reviewing the results of the medical tests, the Applied Kinesiologist confirmed her original diagnosis that a hiatal hernia was the probable cause of her GERD.

Gloria also shared that, during the summer before her recent condition started, she joined an intense exercise program with her friends. One of the exercises commonly done was abdominal crunches. While abdominal exercises done properly have many health benefits, most people tend to do them improperly and end up disrupting the stabilizing muscles of the core area.

The Applied Kinesiologist asked her to describe the exercises. Some involved the usual hands-behind-the-head position while sitting up and down. Another involved lifting the legs during the crunch. This exercise uses the psoas muscle which lies under the abdominals, connects to all the lumbar spinal bones and runs through your groin to connect to the inner thigh. The psoas supports the natural curve of your lumbar spine; whereas the abdominals flex and flatten out the lumbar curve. It is a physiological fact that the psoas muscle and the rectus abdominal muscles or "abs" are antagonistic and, when used together, can create dysfunction. Unfortunately, most abdominal exercises mistakenly involve both simultaneously.

Gait Analysis revealed her taking an obvious shorter stride with her left leg and that her right foot rotated out to the side dramatically more than her left.

The doctor began the examination by functionally muscle testing the left psoas muscle which proved inhibited. The psoas muscle connects to the tendons of the diaphragm. These tendons, comprising the crural part of the diaphragm, form an opening known as the *esophageal hiatus* where the esophagus enters the abdominal cavity. The crural diaphragm also provides a strong sphincter mechanism. This mechanism provides protection against acid reflux. It has appropriately been called the "*external* lower esophageal sphincter."

Additionally, one of the ligaments of the diaphragm (medial arcuate ligament) wraps around the psoas muscle. An imbalance of any of these can lead to an abnormal weakening of the opening of the esophageal hiatus allowing the stomach to slide up beyond the diaphragm. When this happens, the LES also becomes compromised and can cause the reflux of gastric acid or GERD.

The Applied Kinesiologist explained that while traditional medicine often prescribed surgery to correct this condition, it was not necessary in her case. He described the underlying muscular dysfunction which was most likely caused, not by the sausage hero or her diet, but by the extreme nature of her exercise routine that compromised her psoas muscle and led to the weakening of the diaphragm and the resulting hiatus hernia. Through a noninvasive AK treatment regimen, he could restore the muscle function and coax the stomach back down below the diaphragm. Once that was accomplished, her reflux would disappear. Gloria was relieved and agreed to start treatment immediately.

The doctor had Gloria lie on the examination table as he facilitated the left psoas muscle to normal strength through precise manipulation of the Golgi tendon organ at the insertion of the muscle into the hip. Then the doctor elevated the table to a 45-degree position and proceeded to restore the stomach to its proper position beneath the diaphragm. He placed his hands over the epigastric area just below the left border of the ribcage where her stomach had been pushed upward. He performed The Hiatal Hernia Maneuver for five breathing cycles. After the last maneuver, the doctor could feel a release of pressure under his finger—like a cork coming out of a bottle.

After this procedure, Gloria said that she could take a "real breath" for the first time in months. The doctor explained that as her stomach moved back into its normal position, the diaphragm and lungs could then function freely. Once the psoas muscle had regained its proper function, it maintained the position of the diaphragm in relation to the esophageal hiatus and restored its ability to act as a natural barrier to acid reflux.

Furthermore, the AK practitioner explained that this was only the first stage of the treatment. Since Gloria's hernia had been pronounced for a few months, the ligament that attaches the stomach to the diaphragm had become weakened as well. It would take a few months for the ligament to heal and perform its proper function of keeping the stomach in place. Once it was back to normalcy, Gloria would be cured of the hernia and its symptoms.

The healing process would involve some lifestyle changes and follow-up visits to ensure that the stomach remained in position. The doctor instructed Gloria to squat down from the hips when picking items up off the floor and place her foot up onto a stool or stair step to tie her shoes. He recommended that she stop taking her PPI medications and to begin taking a mineral supplement of manganese to help her ligaments to heal. The doctor also suggested drinking water mostly between meals and sipping only a little liquid with meals, since drinking too much with food can lead to reflux symptoms. He also instructed his patient not to lie down after eating. The doctor suggested that she continue with her restricted diet to prevent reflux and allow the esophagus lining to heal; as well as to gargle and drink aloe vera juice twice a day to help speed up the healing process.

Most importantly, Gloria was no longer to perform abdominal crunches during her workout. The doctor taught her a standing, predominately isometric abdominal exercise that she could safely do. The exercise naturally contracts the abdominals and brings the ribcage slightly down toward the pubic bone without impacting on the psoas muscle. He recommended that she do this daily for three sets of 12 repetitions.

When Gloria returned for her second visit, she happily reported that she only felt a slight twinge of heartburn after she ate. The doctor examined her and found that while her psoas muscle remained strong, the stomach had slipped up again. Gloria confessed that she had forgotten to put her foot up, as instructed, to tie her shoes. This simple action had caused the stomach to rise back up again.

The doctor repositioned the stomach and stimulated the weakened ligament of the diaphragm with a Vibracussor®. He then taught Gloria proper diaphragmatic breathing exercises to strengthen her diaphragm muscle, promoting its ability to act as a shield in preventing the recurrence of the hiatal hernia. She returned weekly for the same treatment and experienced no further symptoms. After a month of taking manganese, Gloria switched to taking a balanced multi-mineral supplement that contained manganese and other minerals essential for good ligament, bone, and endocrine health.

Gloria required a total of eight treatments. She kept to her adjusted diet and new exercise regimen. Her hiatal hernia was healed, and all of her symptoms were relieved.

Ileocecal Valve Syndrome

The ileocecal valve (ICV) is critical to intestinal health. It is located just above the appendix at the junction of the *ileum,* the end of your small intestine, and the *cecum* which is a pouch at the beginning of your large intestine (colon). As the cecum becomes distended with food waste, the large intestine signals the sphincter muscle to close the valve to prevent reflux of food meant to be eliminated from the body back into the small intestine where it can enter the bloodstream. This process is called the *ICV cecal distention reflex.*

Ileocecal Valve Syndrome is caused by dysfunction of the ICV, which prevents it from keeping out fecal matter and bacteria from entering the small intestine. This fecal matter is toxic and, if it enters the bloodstream, it can have a wide-ranging impact on the entire body. The symptoms of this condition include constipation, diarrhea, abdominal bloating and pain, inflamed pelvic organs, ovarian pain, prostate problems, severe low back pain, disc swelling, sciatica, edema/swelling in your feet or hands, premenstrual syndrome (PMS), headaches, dizziness, sinus congestion, ringing in the ears, skin problems, fatigue, dark circles under your eyes, and colic in infants.

Because the symptoms are so varied and associated with many conditions, ICV syndrome is often referred to as "the great mimicker" and difficult to diagnose. Traditional medicine treats the most obvious and acute symptoms, often misdiagnosing the fundamental cause. AK specialists are well acquainted with this syndrome and its wide-reaching impact on the body. In fact, since it is so pervasive, it is high on the list of possible sources for a patient's discomfort. Using their unique and exhaustive examination techniques, AK specialists can diagnose Ileocecal Valve Syndrome quickly and treat it more effectively. Once the muscular valve is restored to its proper function, the symptoms usually clear up on their own through the body's natural cleansing mechanisms.

* * *

HENRIETTA, 45, suffered from severe abdominal discomfort for as long as she could remember. After having been promoted to become the highest-ranking female in the financial institution, where she had worked for over 20 years, her level of stress increased. She started to suffer from a variety of additional health issues such as severe abdominal bloating in connection with menstruation, chronic constipation, and lower back pain. Her problems grew worse with each passing day and affected both her work and home life.

Her long-time family doctor could not help her and referred her to a gastroenterologist. He performed a series of tests, including a colonoscopy. The results of the colonoscopy were unremarkable, and the other tests proved inconclusive. Based on her symptoms, the specialist concluded that Henrietta was suffering from Irritable bowel syndrome (IBS), a serious chronic intestinal condition. It is often associated with an excess of bacteria in the colon and exacerbated by stress. He prescribed a series of antibiotics and told her to stay away from any foods that might cause intestinal gas such as broccoli, cabbage, and certain fruits. She also took a laxative for her constipation. She experienced a brief relief from some of the symptoms, but they soon returned in full force. She was so distraught that she was considering taking an antidepressant to help with her anxiety.

As is often the case, Henrietta came to AK through a fellow sufferer. A close friend of her husband noticed that Henrietta was not eating much at a dinner party that they all attended. She looked so uncomfortable that the friend asked her if something was wrong. Henrietta shared her diagnosis of IBS and how miserable she had been. The friend admitted that she, too, was a fellow sufferer and had tried all the treatments. Nothing had worked. Finally, she sought an alternative therapist certified in AK. He went on to relieve the symptoms within six months, and she felt great ever since. Henrietta was wary at first but took the name and number of the specialist. She figured getting a second opinion from an entirely different perspective couldn't hurt.

During the consultation, the doctor reviewed her medical records and listened while she explained her symptoms. She was near tears describing her problem. Gait analysis revealed that she walked with a shorter stride on her right leg. Postural Analysis showed that she was "knock-kneed" as well.

The examination began with manual muscle testing of her right psoas muscle and both sartorius muscles. All three were inhibited, which would explain the shorter right stride and the knock-knees. The sartorius muscle stabilizes the knee and has a neural connection to the adrenal glands that act as the "first-responders" to stress (a possible reason why people's knees knock when they are nervous).

The psoas muscle is instrumental in the initiation of the forward movement of your leg in walking due to its connection to the inside of your thighbone. It connects to a wide range of other tissues, including the mesentery or internal membrane that serves to anchor the intestines to the abdominal wall. The small intestine mesentery has a connection to the ICV as well. An imbalance of the psoas muscles, particularly on the right, can affect the function of the ICV by pulling on the mesenteric connection to the valve.

As the longest muscles in the body, the sartorius muscles often are linked to adrenal general adaptation syndrome (GAS), in conjunction with other secondary conditions related to adrenal stress such as autoimmune diseases. Overproduction of adrenal hormones, namely adrenaline and cortisol can exacerbate ongoing stress levels and impact intestinal health.

The exam continued by having Henrietta engage in Therapy Localization over the area between the umbilicus and the hipbone on the right, near the location of the ileocecal valve. The muscle closely related to the intestines, the tensor fascia lata, became dramatically inhibited with Henrietta's hand over this area when tested. When she gently Challenged the muscle by pulling upward on the area, simulating the *ICV cecal distention reflex,* the muscle regained its normal function. This result indicated a dysfunction in the ICV.

Based on this information, the specialist shared his theory that her condition was not IBS, but Ileocecal Valve Syndrome. He explained the nature of the condition and that it shared many of the symptoms with IBS, leading many medical doctors to misdiagnose a patient with the more serious condition. Since the ICV syndrome is basically a mechanical dysfunction due to pressure from the muscles surrounding the valve itself as well as those inside the intestines, it can be corrected by targeted manipulation. Henrietta was shocked and relieved at this information. The doctor said he could start treatment immediately, and she readily agreed.

First, the doctor manipulated the Golgi tendons organs at their insertion to the hip, returning Henrietta's psoas to normal physiological strength. Having restored the stabilizing function of the psoas muscle, he moved on to the ICV. After about a minute of deep manipulation, a palpable and audible gurgle emanated from the area. Henrietta felt immediate relief from her abdominal pain, and the pressure she had been feeling for months all but disappeared. The doctor instructed her to put some cold water in a Ziploc® bag and place it over her abdominal area for twenty minutes every hour that evening and, if she felt up to it, take an enema to clear out her lower intestine. He advised her to come back in two days.

On her next visit, Henrietta reported that she felt very little pain and that her system seemed to be less impacted. After further ICV manipulation, the doctor recommended that she take the herb rhodiola to help with stress reduction, a probiotic pill to improve her gut microbiome, and an extract of chlorophyll to help soothe and heal the intestinal tissues after the ravages of toxicity they had experienced.

Henrietta required three months of weekly treatments, after which she was completely cured. Her anxiety level had also decreased substantially, now that her intestinal health had been restored.

CHRONIC CONSTIPATION

Chronic constipation is a common condition with far-reaching health implications. Constipation is defined as difficulty in having a bowel movement or having one fewer than three times a week. The National Institute of Diabetes, and Digestive and Kidney Diseases states that constipation is one of the most common digestive problems in the United States affecting approximately 42 million Americans.[30] Reportedly, constipation leads to 6 million doctors' appointments and over 700,000 emergency room visits yearly.[31] This results in $12.7 billion of direct medical costs.[32]

The large intestine is where the unwanted waste of your diet is excreted from your body. However, most people do not realize that, while most of the absorption of nutrients occurs in your small intestine, the majority of the water you drink is absorbed in the large intestine. If you are not properly hydrated, your large intestine or colon will hold on to the unwanted food in an attempt to absorb the last drops of water. This *holding on* and poor diet are the major factors contributing to constipation.

Constipation can be a painful condition leading to abdominal pain, gas and general discomfort. It can also impact the health of the liver. Of the nearly 500 functions of your liver, one of the most important is to detoxify the large intestine. Therefore, because chronic constipation keeps toxic fecal waste in the colon, it can unduly place a strain on your liver and impede its other important functions.

In addition to a lack of water intake, common causes of constipation are dietary deficiencies of fiber and minerals (notably magnesium); lack of exercise; certain medications such as opiates, antacids, antidepressants, and anti-hypertensives; and biomechanical issues such as poor posture and bony misalignment of the pelvic, lumbar, or cranial structures—all of which can lead to neurogenic dysfunction of the nerves that control the large intestine muscles.

* * *

BENGINA, 58, was a seamstress who worked tirelessly at home and at her small shop. She had an optimistic attitude, laughed often, and even played the harmonica while people tried on their newly altered wardrobe. She ate a healthy diet. Her only habitual health flaws were that she never drank water, opting instead for juice and tea, and her bowel movements were infrequent. She would go days, sometimes a week, without a bowel movement. It was uncomfortable, but it never seemed to hold her back from her hectic schedule.

After suffering a mild stroke, her doctor put her on blood thinners; and instead of immediately prescribing a cholesterol-lowering drug, advised her to drink water and include more fiber in her diet in the form of psyllium husk capsules to help with cardiovascular conditions and proper bowel health. Psyllium is a soluble fiber which can reduce the absorption of "bad cholesterol" (LDL) into your bloodstream. However, while she regained her energy, she still suffered from constipation.

Bengina was referred to a gastroenterologist, who ran several tests including an abdominal X-ray, CT scan and, finally, a barium enema which looked for any possible intestinal obstruction. These tests showed that her intestines were severely blocked with stool, but no definitive cause was found. The GI specialist gave a diagnosis of intestinal pseudo-obstruction. This condition acknowledges a severe blockage in the lower intestine from an unknown cause. He prescribed a medication to help move the stool along by causing muscle contractions in the intestines. However, it made her nauseous, so she stopped taking it. Her constipation continued and was now compounded by low back pain.

At first, she just thought the back pain came from sitting too long at her sewing machine. But the pain got so bad that she could hardly sit down for any amount of time. Her doctor suggested she make an appointment with the osteopathic doctor who was affiliated with their medical group for her low back pain.

The osteopathic doctor, who was also certified in AK, read her patient profile and asked Bengina if she had ever felt low back pain before. She said that she always had some low back pain but just disregarded it as part of age-related aches and pains. She asked the doctor why the low back pain was more pronounced now after all this "poking around" in her intestines. She also shared that it wasn't until she had a stroke that she paid much attention to her chronic constipation. In fact, she rarely felt the urge to have a bowel movement at all. The doctor surmised that this could be caused by a weakening and relative paralysis of the smooth muscles in the intestines responsible for pushing food through. This muscle "weakness" could be traced to faulty neural control due to bony misalignments in the lumbar and pelvic area affecting the nerves that control these muscles. The doctor also explained that there is a strong neural correlation between the low back and the abdominal organs.

The doctor noticed immediately on Gait and the Postural Analysis that Bengina was slightly bow-legged and had a severe swayback condition in her low back as if she were leaning slightly backward.

During the examination, AK manual muscle testing revealed inhibition of the tensor fascia lata (TFL) muscles on the sides of her legs, which can lead to bow leggedness due to a lack of outer support of the thigh. He also discovered a fascial shortening of her hamstring muscles caused by sitting for twelve to sixteen hours daily. Applied Kinesiologists have found that these two muscles share common neurogenic function related to the large intestines. This led the doctor to test for and discover an underlying ileocecal valve (ICV) syndrome as well.

The doctor shared his findings with Bengina, who didn't understand what her legs had to do with her bowels; but she trusted the doctor and agreed to start therapy. Treatment consisted of manual manipulation of the ICV, deep medical massage of the TFL muscle, and fascial lengthening with a Vibracussor® over the hamstring muscles. After the treatments, her lower back pain was very much relieved.

When Bengina returned three days later for a follow-up visit, she reported that her low back pain was much better, but she still suffered from constipation. The doctor examined further and found that the large bone of the pelvis (the ilium) was misaligned in a forward position on both sides. Also, her first lumbar vertebra in her low back was misaligned; this misalignment could put undue pressure on the hypogastric nerve, which controls the lower colon, rectum, and sphincters.

The doctor made three spinal manipulations to the lumbar and pelvic bones and again treated the muscles and ICV as in the previous visit. He then instructed Bengina on squatting down every morning to help keep the pelvic bones aligned and open up the rectum by relaxing the puborectalis muscle which would help facilitate bowel movements. Due to chronic tightness in her low back as well as in her ankles and knees, she was unable to achieve this position initially. The doctor told Bengina to keep at it and also advised her to place her feet on a small step stool in front of the toilet to better maintain this natural position when having a bowel movement.

After four months of weekly treatments to her muscles, pelvic and spinal bones, Bengina was able to squat all the way down and rise up without difficulty. The doctor also encouraged her to get up from her sewing machine and move around for ten minutes every hour. These daily exercises, supported by proper hydration, spinal alignment, and increased fiber in her diet, allowed Bengina to have daily bowel movements as well as experience little to no low back pain.

* * *

The GI tract is one of the most complex systems in the body. Traditional medicine often focuses on the biochemical approach relying on antibiotics, laxatives, stool softeners, muscle relaxers, and pain relief medications to relieve symptoms of conditions such as GERD and IBS. Often, surgery is recommended if these medications prove ineffective. As illustrated in the cases above, this protocol doesn't treat the fundamental cause, which is usually a physiological dysfunction of the biomechanics of the system. Applied Kinesiology, with its unique diagnostic and treatment methods, can relieve a wide variety of symptoms and cure people of many of these gastrointestinal problems as well as prevent them from recurring.

11

"HEART" CONDITIONS

As we've seen, AK is about function, movement, and muscles. There are three types of muscles in your body: skeletal, smooth and cardiac. Skeletal muscles are attached to bone and skin and are responsible for the movement of limbs, eyes, tongue, spine, skull, and other body parts. Smooth muscles are found in the walls of hollow organs such as the lower end of the esophagus, stomach, intestines, bladder, blood vessels, lungs, uterus, prostate, and internal muscles of the eye. Cardiac muscle is a specialized form of muscle tissue, with characteristics of skeletal and smooth muscle, found only in the heart.

Cardiac muscle comprises the wall of the heart and is responsible for the muscular contractions that continuously pump blood throughout your body. Unique to cardiac muscle is *auto-rhythmicity,* or the capacity to set its own contraction rhythm. The heart itself has a natural "pacemaker," the sinoatrial node, which does not rely exclusively on the general nervous system to function like other muscles.

The main control of the heart resides in the medulla oblongata, the lowest part of the brain and uppermost part of your spinal cord, which contains an area called the cardio-regulatory center. The nerves that regulate the heart consist of both sympathetic (stimulating) and parasympathetic (relaxing) parts. The sympathetic nervous system acts upon the sinoatrial node to increase the heart rate. The parasympathetic system, through the vagus nerve, works in reverse to slow the heart rate down. Nerves from both pass down from the brain stem (connecting the brain to your spinal cord) to join the cardiac plexus, where they enter the heart itself.

The heart is generally considered the hardest working muscle in your body. It beats about 100,000 times a day and pumps at least 2,000 gallons of blood[33] through the approximately 60,000 miles of blood vessels contained within your body. About the size of your fist, it sits in your chest cavity, surrounded by the sternum (breastbone) and ribcage. The heart is encased in a fibro-serous sac called the pericardium. The pericardium is attached to the sternum and is firmly connected to the central tendon of the diaphragm. This strong encasing protects the heart and lubricates it as it continuously beats. Your heart has four chambers: the right atrium receives blood from the veins and pumps it to the right ventricle, which then sends the blood to the lungs for oxygenation; the left atrium receives this freshly oxygenated blood and sends it to the left ventricle, where it is sent throughout the entire body. Each of these chambers has a valve that opens and contracts to control the blood flow.

Heart disease is the leading cause of death worldwide and represents a collective term for a variety of conditions including heart attacks, coronary artery disease, angina, arrhythmia, valve dysfunction, heart failure, and other conditions. A heart attack, also called a myocardial infarction (MI), occurs when the blood flow to the heart becomes blocked, cutting off oxygen to its muscle. Symptoms such as chest pain or pressure, arm or jaw pain, inexplicable sweating, trouble breathing, and light-headedness are potential signs of a heart attack and should not be ignored.

Like other muscles and organs, your heart is dependent upon many structural factors to maintain its proper function such as regular electrical impulses from the nervous system, optimal blood flow, and the free movement of connected supportive structures. Pathological heart disease is serious and life-threatening and requires medical intervention. However, many conditions can simulate the symptoms of heart disease but arise from the improper functioning of the internal skeletal and muscular structures that surround the heart. Applied Kinesiology's focus on the interconnectivity of the systems in the body can recognize these conditions and avoid unnecessary invasive procedures.

Thoracic Outlet Syndrome

Thoracic outlet syndrome (TOS) occurs when the nerves or blood vessels in your neck and shoulder regions are compressed by surrounding structures such as a rib. The thoracic outlet is a narrow space between your collarbone and first rib located near your lower neck and upper chest where blood vessels, nerves and muscles pass through. It is surrounded by the neck flexor, upper trapezius, and pectoral muscles. Symptoms include pain, numbness, tingling or weakness of the neck, chest, shoulder and/or arm. Cold hands are a frequent complaint due to impaired circulation. Well-known causes of TOS include physical trauma such as car accidents; repetitive sports-related activities (most commonly baseball pitching and basketball shooting); poor posture; pregnancy; and certain anatomical defects, such as having an extra rib.

Treatment generally begins with various medications such as anti-inflammatories, thrombolytics to break up blood clots, or anticoagulants to prevent them. Additionally, exercises and PT to stretch and/or strengthen the chest muscles to restore normal posture in an attempt to relieve compression on the nerves and blood vessels are usually implemented. If these do not help, thoracic outlet decompression surgery to remove structures, such as a rib, may be attempted. Applied Kinesiologists have learned that there are physiological reasons for TOS that are readily corrected without requiring surgery.

* * *

SARAH, 30, was a new mother. Several months after she started breastfeeding, she felt like her chest was tightening up and began to have shooting pains in her arm and chest. Worried that it was a heart attack, she called her pediatrician who told her to go to the ER. Fortunately, after a battery of tests, the doctors ruled out a heart attack. She was released with a referral to a cardiologist to investigate the problem further. After reviewing the test results, the cardiologist suggested that Sarah's chest pains stemmed from a mitral valve prolapse, a condition in which the flaps of the valve that regulates the blood flow from atrium to ventricle don't close properly. This condition can lead to other life-threatening problems and often requires surgery.

It just didn't make sense to Sarah. She was young, had never had any signs or symptoms of heart disease, and didn't have a history of heart problems in her family. She couldn't afford to undergo surgery with a newborn at home. She shared this diagnosis with her pediatrician and general practitioner, both of whom did not agree with it. The pediatrician felt it was, in all likelihood, some kind of musculoskeletal strain and referred her to her personal chiropractor who specialized in AK.

During her initial consultation, Sarah shared that she had never had a heart problem, and this condition started when she started nursing. The doctor asked Sarah to simulate her position when breastfeeding. Like many women, Sarah assumed a position that had her hunch over to cradle the baby while nursing. As she did, she felt the start of the chest pain on her left side. However, when she demonstrated her position when nursing on the right side, she had no pain. The doctor explained that when held in place for an extended period during breastfeeding, the hunched over position put undue pressure on the left chest muscles causing the left shoulder to curl forward. This compromises the thoracic outlet area through which the nerves pass going down the arm—the result is intense pain.

Postural Analysis confirmed that Sarah's left shoulder was noticeably twisted forward compared to her right. Gait Analysis exaggerated this distortion so dramatically that she essentially looked like she was about to throw a punch (a left hook specifically) when her left arm and right leg went forward.

Upon examination, the doctor noted that Sarah's left hand was significantly colder than her right and that her radial pulse on the inside of her wrist was diminished. Sarah's grip, when measured on a Dynamometer, was much weaker on the left—more than to be expected—even though she was right-handed.

AK muscle testing revealed that fascial shortening, concentrated in a specific area deep in her left pectoralis minor muscle, had created a trigger point that impacted the entire left shoulder girdle and chest region. When palpated, pain shot through her chest and down her left arm, simulating what many people might think is a symptom of a heart attack. Further functional muscle testing revealed the pectoralis minor muscle to be strong initially but became inhibited after it was stretched. Additional muscle testing uncovered an inhibition of one of the midback muscles on the left, known as the lower trapezius. Palpation also revealed a restriction of the spinal vertebrae where the lower trapezius muscle originates from on the spine, as well as a severe "locking up" of the joint where the first rib connects to the spine.

All of these factors contributed to the doctor's diagnosis that Sarah was suffering from TOS, a disorder in which blood vessels and nerves become compressed in the space between the first rib and the collarbone in the front of the chest. Applied Kinesiologists and other functional medicine specialists have found that the most common cause of TOS is a myofascial trigger point in the pectoralis minor muscle. When TOS occurs on the left side, the symptoms of tightening in the chest and shooting pains along the left arm often are mistaken for a heart condition. Diagnosis of this painful condition often eludes traditional cardiac tests and can be misidentified as originating with the heart itself, as in Sarah's case.

Sarah was understandably relieved when the doctor shared his diagnosis with her. It confirmed her confusion regarding the cardiologist's evaluation and her pediatrician's concerns about his diagnosis. She asked the doctor if she could solve the problem simply by adjusting her position while breastfeeding. Unfortunately, since the pain was so pronounced, it indicated that the TOS had progressed to the point that it required treatment to relieve it. Once that was accomplished, adjusting her position would help prevent it from recurring.

The treatment involved several procedures in getting the muscles functioning properly and relieving the pressure on the nerves and blood vessels within the thoracic outlet. It began with manipulation of the lower midback muscle by stimulating the nerve endings known as Golgi tendon organs. By specifically applying pressure in the proper direction to the ends of a muscle, an Applied Kinesiologist can alter the nerve impulses via the feedback mechanism of the Golgi tendon organs in that muscle and restore normal function to it immediately.

Once the middle back muscle was functioning properly, the doctor proceeded to restore normal motion to Sarah's spine with a spinal adjustment, followed by another precise manipulation to the first rib to open up the thoracic outlet. Finally, to release the compression on the nerves and blood vessels that traverse through the thoracic outlet, the doctor performed a fascial manipulation of the pectoral and shoulder muscles, specifically the pectoralis minor. Using a cold-and-stretch procedure, the doctor applied an ice pack over the area and proceeded to stretch the shortened muscle to eliminate the trigger point. Sarah felt relief almost immediately.

To follow up on the strengthening process, the doctor instructed Sarah how to perform the Door Stretch to open up her ribs, shoulders, and chest. The Door Stretch is a procedure in which you wedge your elbows and forearms in an open doorway, slightly above your shoulders. One foot is placed in front of the other, and you gently lean forward to stretch out your chest muscles (as well as the calf and groin muscles on the back leg) for 30 seconds. Switch legs and repeat. The doctor also instructed Sarah to get a light dumbbell (5 lbs.) and do one-arm rowing exercises to strengthen the strained lower trapezius muscle. Finally, doctor and patient found a less stressful position for Sarah to nurse on her left side.

After six weeks of treatments to maintain proper shoulder biomechanics and spinal alignment along with home exercises and stretches, Sarah was completely cured of her shooting pains—with no signs of cold hands, arm weakness, or "heart" problems.

Heart Palpitations

Heart palpitations are the sensations that your heart is fluttering, missing a beat, or pounding. While heart palpitations are worrisome, they are usually harmless. They can be due to emotional stress, certain medications and other drugs, excessive caffeine, pregnancy, hormonal imbalances, dehydration, abnormal electrolyte levels, and fatigue. More serious causes include other heart problems such as arrhythmias (irregular heartbeat), heart defects, and heart diseases. Atrial fibrillations are reported to be the most common form of heart arrhythmia and one of the leading conditions that lead to strokes—the second leading cause of death in the world. Most of these conditions are treated with drugs such as blood thinners, beta blockers, and statins; as well as a surgical procedure known as cardiac ablation.

Functional medicine specialists recognize that your heart does not sit alone in a vacuum, but rather within the thoracic cavity where it is surrounded by a protective ribcage and separated from your abdominal cavity by your diaphragm muscle. Any biomechanical aberrations regarding these structures can alter the intrathoracic pressure within your chest and put undue stress on your heart. These problems are usually *functional* and are usually *fixable.*

* * *

JENNY, 62, enrolled in a yoga class to help relieve her chronic low back pain. After a month, she was having serious heart palpitations, shortness of breath, and chest pains in addition to her low back pain. Since she developed her symptoms after enrolling in yoga class, it was logical to assume that some kind of physiological trauma related to the stretching process was the underlying cause of her problem. She stopped going to yoga, but the pains continued.

Concerned, she visited her doctor who took blood tests and an electrocardiogram. None of the results indicated any kind of heart condition. However, since the pains continued, she suggested Jenny consult with a cardiologist After reviewing the tests, the specialist rendered a diagnosis of atrial fibrillation or irregular heartbeats. He recommended a host of treatments including blood thinners and beta blockers, and an invasive procedure called cardiac ablation wherein a doctor inserts a thin tube through a patient's blood vessels to scar or destroy the tissue in the heart that is causing the abnormal heart rhythms.

As Jenny had no history of heart disease and all her tests were negative for any pathology in her heart, she didn't understand how the doctor had diagnosed her with this condition. When she shared the doctor's recommendations with her brother, who was a chiropractor, he agreed with her skepticism about the diagnosis. Believing it was in some way linked to her yoga experience, he referred Jenny to a colleague who specialized in AK.

When Jenny entered the doctor's consultation room, she was in obvious distress. She shared that her chests pains had begun when she started her yoga class, as well as her concern about the diagnosis of the cardiologist. The doctor asked her to describe the yoga exercises she had performed and then proceeded to review all of her tests. He told Jenny that nothing in the test results supported the diagnosis she had received and suspected that there was nothing wrong with her heart—her symptoms might be functional in nature.

Postural Analysis revealed that Jenny had an increased curve in her low back which seemed to cause her abdominal area to bulge slightly. Gait Analysis displayed the same excessive lumbar (low back) curvature, so much so that she looked as if she was leaning backward and leading with her stomach as she walked.

The doctor had her sit on the examination table and listened with a stethoscope to her heart over all four valves. They all sounded within normal limits. She then lied face up on the table, and he began to palpate the temporal-sphenoidal (TS) line reflex points on both sides of her head. The doctor felt two distinct nodules at the points that correspond to her abdominal (stomach) muscles and the adductor (groin) muscles. The doctor asked Jenny to sit up so that he could manually muscle test her abdominals and adductors. Both muscles were severely inhibited, as evidenced by the fact that the patient could barely sit up for the test and was unable to hold her ankles together to test the groin muscles.

After testing the abdominals, Jenny lay back on the table. As she did so, she complained of heart flutters. The doctor listened; sure enough, he could hear an erratic heartbeat. The doctor assured

Jenny that this reaction was to be expected when a patient lies down, especially after having tested a dysfunctional abdominal muscle in conjunction with what the doctor suspected was causing Jenny's irregular heart rhythms. Upon further examination, Jenny's weak abdominals and adductor muscles of the groin were apparently due to a slight misalignment of her pubic bones. This was confirmed when Jenny Therapy Localized the pubic symphysis, the joint connecting the two ramus bones of the pelvis. This is commonly known as symphysis pubic dysfunction (SPD). While this usually creates problems in the pelvic region, in Jenny's case it created a neural dysfunction of her abdominal muscles and destabilized the position of the stomach and ribcage as well—resulting in a *hiatal hernia*.

You may remember that a hiatal hernia is a syndrome wherein the stomach slips too close to the diaphragm impeding its natural movement and limiting ribcage motion. This can result in a buildup of pressure in the thoracic cavity. The outer covering of your heart (pericardium) connects to the central tendon of your diaphragm, and any diaphragmatic disturbances can affect heart mechanics. Depending on the individual, it can cause, among other things, heart palpitations. The doctor asked Jenny if she had any reflux symptoms. She replied that she did, but they were infrequent and not severe.

The doctor also used Pulse Point Analysis and found what acupuncturists diagnose as an energy blockage within the *alarm point* of the heart meridian. This acupuncture point is called the "Gateway to the Heart" and sits just below the breastbone.

The doctor shared his diagnosis that Jenny was suffering from a hiatal hernia, which caused increased pressure in the chest and affected the normal rhythms of the heart. While relieved that it wasn't a heart condition, Jenny was concerned about the hernia. She had heard that this condition also required surgery. The doctor said that her hernia resulted from the effects of the dysfunctional abdominal muscles as a consequence of SPD and would not require surgery.

The doctor surmised that Jenny "dove into yoga" a bit too strenuously and *strained* several of her muscles. She did not do enough to *sprain* a joint, but she created strenuous tension in several muscles to the degree that the Golgi tendon receptors perceived it as enough to warrant their "shutting down the muscles" to protect them. These chronically *strained* muscles were probably the cause of Jenny's chronic low back issues to begin with. In all likelihood, had she started her yoga more gently and avoided the erroneous *no pain no gain* mantra, which she mentioned she adhered to, she may have avoided her lower back problems and would definitely not have strained the muscles leading to her diaphragm and, subsequent, irregular heartbeat symptoms.

The doctor began treatment by gently realigning the pelvic bones by having Jenny squeeze a tennis ball between her knees. She was startled when the bones made an audible "thunk" as the bones shifted back into place. The doctor then manipulated the Golgi tendon organs (GTO) at the pubic bone, as well as the lower ribcage, to restore the normal physiological tone and function to the abdominals. He then performed the same technique for the adductor muscles. With the abdominal and the pelvic muscles now functioning properly, the doctor addressed the hiatal hernia. After manipulating her stomach into its proper position beneath the diaphragm, Jenny felt relief from the chest pressure she had been feeling. Lastly, the doctor treated the heart meridian alarm point with a tei-shin, an acupuncture-stimulating device that does not pierce the skin.

To restore the ribcage and diaphragm to their normal relationship during the breathing cycle, the doctor administered spinal adjustments to the vertebrae where the diaphragm connects in the lumbar region and then taught Jenny the Door Stretch as well as The Wall Stretch. In the latter maneuver, placing the back of your head, hips and heels against the wall, you bring your arms up in front of you, then back toward the wall until the back of your hand touches the wall as you take a deep breath in. Essentially, you are opening up your chest and entire ribcage like an accordion. Jenny was instructed to do this exercise for ten repetitions three times a day, followed by the Door Stretch.

After several treatments to resolve the hernia and ensure the proper alignment of the patient's pelvis, her "heart" symptoms disappeared completely as well as her chronic low back pain. Jenny returned to her yoga classes with a new mindset to stay within her limits so that she would not injure her muscles and joints again.

Slipping Rib Syndrome

Slipping rib syndrome is a condition where your rib(s) slips from its usual position. This little-known and often overlooked problem frequently occurs when you happen to take a breath and bend or twist in a manner that causes a rib to subluxate and slip out of alignment. Symptoms include sharp pain, popping or clicking sounds, difficulty breathing, a palpable lump, and chest pain. Treatments include hot and cold compresses, anti-inflammatory drugs, rest, and PT exercises. Inexplicably, the standard therapeutic protocol for slipping rib syndrome does not include manual manipulation of the *slipped rib* back into proper alignment.

This condition is believed to be rare and to predominately occur with the lower ribs. However, Applied Kinesiologists find slipping rib syndrome to be a common occurrence and that it can affect any rib. Patients' complaints range from a sharp pain that feels like "someone is stabbing me in the back" to a myriad of heart and breathing problems.

* * *

GLEN, 32, was a journalist who was working diligently to meet a deadline for his first book-length project. He was not sleeping much and drinking eight cups of coffee a day to keep up the frenetic pace. One day, after taking a break from writing, he started doing some pushups when his phone rang. He looked up quickly and collapsed onto the floor. He attempted to get up and felt lightheaded and nauseous, then fell back down onto the floor and felt a sharp pain in the left side of his chest and back. He had been lying there for half an hour, unable to get up due to vertigo and chest pains, when his wife found him. She called an ambulance and informed their family doctor.

The emergency room doctors noted that Glen was in respiratory distress, and his blood pressure was high. They took chest X-rays that showed no pulmonary disease, as well as blood tests which only revealed a slightly elevated total cholesterol level. An EKG of his heart function showed two minor abnormalities: sinus arrhythmia, an irregularity in the heart rhythm; and a bi-fascicular block in nerve impulses to both right and left ventricles, which impacts the flow of blood through them. While the doctors did not think these findings were life-threatening, Glen was admitted for observation. His condition remained stable, and he was released the following day. The doctors recommended that he consult with a cardiologist for further evaluation. At home, his dizziness and nausea subsided, but Glen was still barely able to move without severe chest pain and his heart pounding.

Two days later, Glen visited with the cardiologist. The doctor examined him and took a sonogram. The results were normal, despite the pain he was experiencing. Glen was sent for an Electron Beam Tomography (EBT) heart scan to assess if an artery might be blocked with plaque buildup by measuring calcium deposits in the coronary artery; these results were also normal. The cardiologist then recommended that Glen wear a portable Holter heart monitor for 24 hours. The results were normal and only revealed a slight arrhythmia. This being the only abnormal finding, the cardiologist diagnosed his condition as ventricular fibrillation, or a dysfunction in the way the heart pumps blood.

The cardiologist prescribed a statin drug to lower the cholesterol levels to avoid blockage to arteries, along with a beta-blocker. Beta-blockers block the effects of epinephrine secreted from the adrenal (stress) glands which otherwise increase the heart rate, helping it to beat more slowly and with less force. They are used to manage abnormal heart rhythms, protect the heart from a second heart attack, and lower blood pressure. The doctor also wrote a prescription for Glen to go for a coronary angiogram, an X-ray test where a catheter is inserted into an artery in the groin and injected with dye to evaluate the general heart function.

Glen did not feel comfortable with the diagnosis and additional invasive testing. He consulted with his longtime family physician, who was also certified in AK. The doctor knew Glen's medical history and reviewed all the results of the tests that his patient had taken. As the results and diagnosis didn't seem to explain Glen's continuing chest pain and heart palpitations, the physician examined him using AK techniques.

During the consultation, Glen shared that he had been extremely stressed before the incident about meeting a deadline to complete his book. In describing the incident, Glen related that he had heard several "popping sounds" while doing push-ups before lifting his head up when the phone rang.

Postural and Gait analysis did not reveal any obvious issues. However, the doctor noted that Glen had a limited range of head motion, and his breathing became a bit shallow when he looked up during the range of motion studies. Any movement caused him to feel heart palpitations. The physician took out a tape measure and measured Glen's chest and ribcage when he took a deep breath. The average ribcage should expand above 4 cm when you take a deep breath in; Glen's only expanded 2 cm. This diminished expansion indicated that there might be some dysfunction in the chest-ribcage-diaphragm relationship.

The doctor began his examination by palpating the serratus anterior and pectoral muscles of the chest and found them to be markedly in spasm. When he palpated over the left side of the chest over the junction of where the fifth rib connects to the breastbone, Glen winced in pain. The doctor then went around to the back and got the same reaction during palpation. Glen Therapy Localized the two areas of the 5th rib's connection points as well as the cervical spine; both were positive and created a muscular disturbance upon functional muscle testing (FMT). Again, when the doctor pressed on the points over the front and back of Glen's ribcage, they consistently sent a piercing pain throughout his chest.

After this examination, the doctor diagnosed Glen with Slipping Rib Syndrome not a dysfunction of the heart itself. He explained what he thought might have happened when Glen heard the phone ring, looked up and fell flat to the floor directly onto his chest—he dislodged a rib causing severe chest and back pain and compromised the natural movement of the entire rib cage. This dislodgement resulted in increased pressure on the chest cavity which affects the pericardium (heart covering), the sternum and diaphragm. Also, when Glen looked up, his neck bones became misaligned; disrupting the phrenic nerve that controls the movement of the diaphragm. This physiological disruption of neural control resulted in labored breathing and increased intrathoracic pressure. All these factors impacted the normal function of the heart and caused dizziness, weakness, and pain.

Under normal circumstances, Glen might not have suffered such drastic effects from his fall. He might have just had a slight bruise instead. However, because he was so stressed, sleep deprived, and overstimulated by caffeine, his system—particularly his heart—were vulnerable to this kind of condition. His body remained out of alignment, which resulted in his overall weakness and continued chest pains. To cure him of this condition, the doctor would need to restore his system to proper alignment and strength.

Treatment began with chiropractic adjustments to the cervical spine and the front and back of the left side of Glen's ribcage along with percussion therapy over the ribs, pectoral muscles, diaphragm and the heart itself. When Glen left, his symptoms were greatly diminished. On the second visit, Glen reported that he continued to feel better. The doctor measured his ribcage and found that it now expanded to 4 cm. Although Glen still felt weak, the severe chest pain was relieved, and the heart palpitations were less pronounced. However, there remained residual pain over the ribcage. The doctor had his patient do a taste test of a high-quality magnesium supplement. When the pain decreased significantly, it was a clear sign that magnesium would help to relieve his muscle spasms. The doctor instructed Glen to start taking a magnesium supplement.

The doctor then adjusted the ribs and showed Glen one of six different rib mobilizing exercises to facilitate rehabilitation of the ribcage and the sternum in the front and the thoracic spine in the back. These movements increase the pliability of the ribcage, thoracic spine, and diaphragm by simulating the natural motion of the ribs during activities such as breathing, walking, bending, lifting, reaching, and throwing.

Glen had seven treatments in total and was back at his desk writing without pain. He does his rib mobilizing exercises three times a day; he is getting more sleep and has learned to take a pause in his day to slow down and spend some time meditating. He has no more than three cups of coffee a day and drinks more water. Although a little later than he wanted, Glen published his first book and is onto his next one in a less manic and far more peaceful pace.

* * *

Chest pain or shooting pains down the arm can be frightening. Most people are quick to jump to the conclusion that these symptoms indicate a heart problem. However, conditions that appear to be heart-related often are not. Traditional medical doctors and specialists are trained to target heart dysfunction when these symptoms occur without taking into consideration the general biomechanics of the entire thoracic system. While it is crucial to rule out heart pathology first, since heart problems can cause chest pain; it is also prudent to understand that structural chest problems can cause heart symptoms.

AK is attuned to the various kinematic factors that can cause symptoms usually associated with heart dysfunction but come from another source. Applied Kinesiology testing and treatments are a valuable adjunct to help find the underlying cause of conditions that seem "heart-related" and cure them.

12

HORMONE IMBALANCES

Hormones are specialized chemical messengers that play a large part in determining our mood, energy levels, sleep patterns, metabolism, sexual function, and physical makeup. About 50 different hormones are circulating in the human body, and most are produced by the various glands that make up our endocrine system. These include the pineal, hypothalamus, pituitary, thyroid, parathyroid, thymus, pancreas, adrenal, and sex glands.

As in every other system in the body, diet plays an important role in maintaining healthy levels of hormones. For instance, your pineal, hypothalamus and pituitary glands need high-quality proteins to produce hormones. The adrenal cortex and sex glands (ovaries and testes) make their respective hormones from the fats and oils you include in your diet. Vitamins and minerals contribute to the production of hormones as well.

Similar to other organs such as your stomach, intestines, and heart, your endocrine glands can be influenced by the complex interrelationships between neural, circulatory, and musculo-skeletal systems that surround them. Dysfunction in any of these systems often causes hormonal imbalances which can affect our overall health.

Unlike traditional medicine which attempts to "fix" conditions linked to hormones by introducing synthetic hormones into the body in an attempt to "balance" the system, AK seeks to find the fundamental cause of the imbalance and help the body restore it naturally through physiological adjustment and nutritional advice. The origin of many conditions linked to hormone imbalances such as insomnia, weight gain, depression, anxiety, chronic infections, autoimmune conditions, diabetes, weak bones, pain, fatigue, menstrual irregularities, and sexual dysfunction can be diagnosed precisely and treated effectively without artificial drugs and invasive procedures.

Adrenal Fatigue Syndrome

Your adrenal glands, commonly known as the "stress glands," are two triangular shaped organs that sit on top of your kidneys in the middle of your low back just below your ribs. One layer of renal fascia (Gerota) covers both the kidneys and the adrenals, and another separates them from each other. The upper portion of your adrenal glands rests on the diaphragm and is also connected to the tendon of the diaphragm by the renal fascia.

Your adrenal glands produce several different hormones and are divided into two distinct zones: the medulla and the cortex. Despite their categorization as a single glandular organ, the two parts of the gland are functionally distinct. The inner part of the adrenal gland, the medulla, makes hormones called catecholamines such as adrenaline—the "fight or flight" hormone. The outer aspect overlying the medulla is the adrenal cortex, which produces three types of steroid-based hormones: aldosterone, which regulates blood pressure; cortisol, which regulates the immune system; and androgens, which help regulate sex organs. The proper balance of all four of these important hormones contributes to the general health of the body.

The medulla part of the adrenal gland helps the body react to stress. This stress response process is well documented in what is known as the general adaptation syndrome (GAS). It manifests in three distinct stages: the *alarm stage*, which gives you a burst of energy in response to a particular situation or traumatic event; the *resistance stage*, where your body resists or adapts to continuing stress; and the *exhaustion stage,* wherein your body's physical resources have been compromised and require restoration. The third stage can be the most dangerous to your health and may lead to Adrenal Fatigue Syndrome (AFS), a condition in which the adrenal gland becomes unable to keep up with the needs of the body to manage stress.

Adrenal Fatigue Syndrome is difficult to diagnose and treat because it can affect so many systems simultaneously. Many of the symptoms of AFS, such as fatigue, abdominal weight gain, chronic pain and inflammation, depression, hypoglycemia, nervousness, brain fog, allergies, reduced sex drive, severe PMS, tendency to tremble when stressed (especially at the knees), lightheadedness when standing, fainting episodes, and unexplained loss of scalp hair, could mistakenly be attributed to a variety of other conditions. Some doctors believe that AFS is associated with a more specific condition known as adrenal insufficiency, which *can* be diagnosed through appropriate blood tests that measure the levels of adrenal hormones.

There are two basic blood tests to assess adrenal gland function. One involves testing for cortisol levels. An unnaturally high or low level of cortisol indicates some kind of adrenal gland dysfunction. However, cortisol levels rise and fall throughout the day, so a single blood test may not be effective for diagnosis. Instead, multiple samples need to be taken at different times to make a complete evaluation with strict comparisons to the reference ranges obtained at the same time the blood sample is drawn.

The other blood test, the *adrenal stimulation test,* measures cortisol levels before and after stimulation of the adrenal glands. For this test, the cortisol level is measured, and then you are injected with a synthetic form of adrenocorticotropic hormone (ACTH), a hormone made by the pituitary gland that stimulates the adrenal glands to make cortisol. After 45 minutes, the blood cortisol level is measured again to see if the adrenal glands have produced more cortisol in response to the ACTH. Failure of your blood cortisol levels to rise suggests adrenal gland malfunction.

However, these blood tests can be inconclusive. Except in the case of severe glandular diseases such as adrenal tumors, Cushing's syndrome (hypercortisolism) or Addison's disease (primary adrenal insufficiency), blood tests often are not precise enough to reveal AFS. This is because each person's body manifests AFS differently. It is not uncommon for the diagnosis, based solely upon these blood tests, to be inaccurate.

Rather than relying upon the fluctuating cortisol levels in the blood, AK focuses on the functional integrity of the fascia, muscles and nervous system that can affect the adrenal glands. Dysfunctions in one or more of these systems can be detected by AK's principal diagnostic tool of FMT. It reveals whether there is a physiological problem outside the adrenal glands that may interfere with their production of hormones. By isolating the underlying cause of the problem, the diagnosis of AFS becomes clear and allows the doctor to treat it effectively.

* * *

KATHY, a 24-year-old computer graphics designer, became concerned when her hair began thinning. At first, it was just a few extra hairs in her hairbrush. But as time progressed, the loss became more dramatic, with clumps of hair falling out each day. Panicked, Kathy sought help from her general doctor, a dermatologist, a nutritionist, and an endocrinologist. She received all the usual blood tests and examinations, which ruled out any serious pathology such as cancer, tumors, skin disease, or allergic reactions—the most common causes of extreme hair loss. However, while the doctors all suspected some kind of hormonal imbalance, none of the tests showed anything conclusive, and the fundamental source of her condition still remained undiagnosed.

Within a few months, Kathy was nearly completely bald and had taken to wearing a wig. She became depressed and stressed about the loss of her hair. Some people inquired whether she was struggling through chemo treatments for cancer, which added to her overall feeling of despair. Both her social and work life suffered.

To make matters worse, Kathy began to experience headaches, neck and jaw tightness and low back pain. One of her coworkers suggested a doctor of chiropractic specializing in AK who had helped her and several other people she knew with these tension-related physical problems. Desperate to get some relief from her condition, Kathy made an appointment.

After reading the detailed patient profile and reviewing her blood tests, the doctor inquired when her hair loss began. Kathy confided that her mother and older sister constantly *guilted* her about moving away to New York City. Adding to her anxiety were her feelings about being able to be successful in her highly competitive field. Her job was hectic but fulfilling, and she loved her little apartment; yet, she was anxious all the time. When she spoke about her situation, the doctor noticed that her jaw tightened, a strong indication that she probably suffered from temporomandibular joint disorder (TMJD), along with bruxism—the involuntary grinding of teeth.

He asked about her headaches and her neck, jaw and low back pains. Kathy related that she was under a great deal of emotional pressure due to the unexplained loss of almost all of her hair. Kathy removed her wig to show her nearly completely bald scalp. None of the doctors she consulted were able to find the cause of her problem. She said her energy levels were so low that she needed, "three cups of coffee just to feel tired." However, while she felt exhausted all the time, she also felt stressed out. Sleep did nothing to help her fatigue. The additional pain added to her stress.

Her medical history indicated that in addition to her hair loss, fatigue, tension headaches, and other pains, Kathy suffered from lightheadedness and sensitivity to light (wearing sunglasses during the interview). She went on to relate that, of all the places where she felt fatigued, she noticed it in her legs specifically—which felt heavy and weak—and that her neck and back felt "super tight."

The doctor recognized that Kathy was suffering from three well-documented functional indicators for adrenal gland dysfunction. They are:

Ragland's Sign. When there is dysfunction of your adrenal glands, they do not properly secrete enough of the catecholamines to regulate abdominal blood flow. This can cause blood pressure to drop to the extent that your body will not compensate for a change in position, such as sitting up from a horizontal position or standing from a sitting position, preventing blood from properly going up to your head and resulting in temporary lightheadedness. This decrease in blood pressure upon arising is also known as orthostatic hypotension.

Arroyo's Sign. The cortex (outer part) of the adrenal gland produces aldosterone that helps regulate mineral balance. If the cortex is not functioning properly, a mineral imbalance occurs that affects the ability of the muscles to work properly. This includes the tiny sphincter muscles of the eye's pupils, which open and constrict to adapt to varying degrees of light. If the pupils are unable to contract when exposed to light, a person will have an abnormal and often painful sensitivity to light.

Rogoff's Sign. Any functional issue involving the muscles at the juncture of the upper lumbar spine and ribcage which are connected to the diaphragm can affect the adrenal glands. Also, the skin mechanoreceptors related to the adrenal glands are located at this junction. If they are compromised due to muscle or adrenal dysfunction, they can become congested and tender to the touch—this is known as a positive Rogoff's sign.

Since Kathy presented with all three of these indicators—lightheadedness, sensitivity to light, and back tightness—the doctor suspected that her problem might be AFS. Postural and Gait Analysis revealed some inner knee instability and a flattening of the lumbar curve, both attributable to a dysfunction of the sartorius—a muscle located in the thigh that runs from the pelvis to the knee. Applied Kinesiologists have empirically found the sartorius to be one of the muscles intimately related to adrenal function, apparently due to their direct involvement with various adrenaline-related activities.

The doctor brought Kathy to the examination room. As Kathy lay face up on the table, the doctor proceeded to test both of her sartorius muscles manually. They were so severely dysfunctional that she could barely position the muscle to comply with the testing procedure. This finding would explain why her legs felt heavy and weak.

The doctor palpated the back of her neck and felt severe tension from what is sometimes called "tech neck," caused by continually looking at computer screens and other devices. The doctor applied pressure to the back of Kathy's neck; she winced and said that she could feel pain shoot up into her head and behind her eye. He also palpated her skull and found it equally tight, as if she were wearing a hat three sizes too small 24/7.

Based on the description, physiological symptoms, and this examination, the doctor diagnosed Kathy as suffering from AFS caused by prolonged stress. He explained that adrenal fatigue can cause lack of energy, muscle pain and tightness, depression, and extreme hair loss. According to her blood tests, the two hormones linked to healthy hair growth: testosterone and dehydroepiandrosterone (DHEA) were deficient in her system and probably had been even before she started to notice her hair loss and other symptoms. Deficiency of these two hormones, which are produced by the adrenal cortex, often leads to hair loss, particularly in women.

Kathy was stunned. She knew she had been under stress, but she had no idea that it could have such a dramatic effect on her. The Applied Kinesiologist explained that the effects of chronic stress are cumulative. As the stress builds, it can cause functional damage gradually to the fascia and nerves vital to the proper function of the adrenal glands. As her emotional stress grew, so did the seriousness of her symptoms, including her hair loss. Her adrenal glands just couldn't keep up. The doctor explained that they would need to work to restore the function of her adrenal glands. Once restored, her symptoms—including her hair loss—would resolve over time.

Kathy's treatment began with deep percussion therapy, as well as an osteopathic manipulation technique to the fascia covering the adrenal gland and the connecting diaphragm and kidneys, followed by stimulation to the skin mechanoreceptors over the junction of the spine and the lower ribcage. These mechanical corrections would free the adrenal glands to begin to function normally.

Next, the Applied Kinesiologist surmised that, in addition to her hormone deficiency, the other contributing factor to her hair loss was that she held most of her stress in her neck just under the skull. This restriction would interfere with the blood flow and lymphatic drainage of her scalp, which could affect the health of her hair follicles. Chiropractic adjustments and trigger point release therapy restored the normal motion of the neck and skull by relieving tension. The doctor then employed specific medical massage techniques to relieve the tension of the spindle cells of the muscles of her skull (specifically the occipitofrontalis muscle) and jaw (temporalis muscle) and manipulated several of her cranial bones manually. Finally, he used a Vibracussor® to increase circulation and drainage of her scalp.

The doctor recommended that she drink more water and cut back on her caffeine; since it is a stimulant, it can add stress to the recuperating adrenal glands. Additionally, the Applied Kinesiologist taught Kathy how to breathe more slowly, using her diaphragm, to better cope with stress and helping maintain the fascial corrections to her diaphragm, adrenals, and kidneys. He suggested that she take some herbal supplements: *rehmannia* as a tonic for her adrenal glands and for its reputed benefits in helping people with autoimmune conditions and hair loss; *skullcap* (scutellaria lateriflora) to calm the nervous system and help her recover from anxiety; and *gotu kola*, "the herb of longevity," to improve circulation to her head, brain and scalp.

Finally, the doctor referred Kathy to a dentist who also specialized in AK manual muscle testing procedures to address her TMJD and help support the muscular corrections made to Kathy's tight jaw muscles.

Kathy came in for biweekly treatments to help the tension in her neck, head, and jaw, as well as to continue releasing the fascial covering over the adrenal glands and improving the function of her sartorius muscles. After a month of treatments, Kathy felt a profound relief from her exhaustion, as well as her neck and lower back pain. The dentist had cured her of the TMJD, further removing tension from her system. The tension headaches, lightheadedness, and sensitivity to light were resolved as well. Within four months, she began to notice hair starting to grow back. After a year of treatments and supplements, Kathy went on to regrow all of her hair and continues to manage her stress productively.

DIABETES

Diabetes is a condition that occurs when your blood sugar (glucose) becomes habitually too high. Diabetes affects 420,000,000 people worldwide.[34] The International Diabetes Federation projects a 50% increase by 2045 to 629,000,000 people.[35] It is the most common endocrine disease in the US with more than 100,000,000 Americans (nearly 30% of the population) harboring diabetes or prediabetes.[36] Over time, people with chronic high blood sugar can develop problems such as heart disease, strokes, nerve damage, kidney problems, eye conditions, dental disorders, and foot problems. Common warning signs of diabetes include increased hunger and thirst, dry mouth, frequent urination or urinary infections, fatigue, blurred vision, headaches, and unexplained weight changes.

The pancreas is about six inches long and looks like a tadpole with a head, body, and tail. It sits behind the stomach and in front of your spine and is the only gland in your body that is both an endocrine gland (makes hormones) and an exocrine gland (secretes digestive enzymes). It produces enzymes that combine with bile (a liquid made by your liver) to digest food, which is called the exocrine function. It also works to balance your blood sugar by making the hormones insulin and glucagon, which is called the endocrine function. The pancreatic cells that make insulin are called the Islets of Langerhans.

People develop diabetes when the pancreas does not manufacture enough of the hormone insulin to control the distribution of glucose in the system or when the body becomes resistant to the insulin produced.

There are two main categories of diabetes: types 1 and 2. Type 1 diabetes is an autoimmune problem wherein your immune system attacks the islet cells and renders them unable to make insulin. This is the more serious of the two, and people who suffer from this type require regular injections of insulin to maintain their glucose levels and have special diets that restrict the intake of foods high in starch and sugar. Type 1 tends to be more common in children and adolescents and requires lifelong management of insulin and diet.

Type 2 occurs when the body does not make enough insulin or becomes resistant to it. Many lifestyle factors contribute to the development of *insulin resistance* in your body and can lead to Type 2 diabetes. While this is commonly called adult-onset diabetes, it is occurring—in increasing numbers—in younger people as childhood obesity, poor nutrition, and inactivity become more prevalent. It is well established that poor diet, obesity and lack of exercise are contributing factors to Type 2 diabetes. Experts explain that these factors make your body more refractory to the effects of insulin. Also, a lack of exercise can cause your muscle cells to lose their sensitivity to insulin, potentially resulting in a rise in blood sugar levels.

Like the other organs and glands in your body, the pancreas responds to stimuli from signals produced by "receptors." Receptors are specialized cells that respond to change. There are external receptors that receive stimuli from the five senses and internal receptors that pick up on the state of your organs, blood pressure, joints, muscles, and posture. When any significant change occurs, receptors send electrical impulses through the nervous system that cause the body to adapt and compensate. If the changes are too great or too frequent, organs and glands can be overstimulated and shut down, producing dysfunction and disease. This is particularly true for the pancreas which, along with the tongue and the gut, has its own taste receptors that can actually *sense* when you are eating sugar and need insulin to be released into the bloodstream to maintain healthy glucose levels. According to new research, *pancreatic receptor dysfunction* might be an additional factor in the increasing prevalence of diabetes.

Because receptors are physiological mechanisms that affect the functionality of our body, AK's unique use of FMT offers *receptor-based treatments* which focus on the various receptors that influence your pancreas and include joint, muscle and skin manipulations. In conjunction with attention to diet and lifestyle, these treatments can prevent and cure the underlying imbalances in pancreatic function which often are the root causes of diabetes.

* * *

GARY, 65, was a machinist all his life. His job was physically demanding and kept him fit. He had always enjoyed relatively good health and never went to doctors. When he retired, he settled into a more sedentary life. However, while his physical activity changed, his diet had not. He had a strong sweet tooth and ate mostly processed foods. As a result, he had slowly packed on the pounds. A few years into his retirement, he hadn't been feeling himself. He was tired all of the time, developed a burning pain in his left shoulder, and had to urinate frequently.

He visited a medical doctor who ran a series of blood tests which revealed that his glucose levels were consistently nearly double the healthy median. Given his other symptoms, the doctor diagnosed him with Type 2 diabetes. He recommended that Gary lose weight, start walking three miles a day, change his diet to include no sweets and more vegetables, and get a home glucose monitor to check his glucose levels regularly. Over the next few months, Gary took great pains to alter his eating habits and exercise. He managed to lose some weight, but his heightened blood glucose level and shoulder pain persisted. His doctor was concerned that his diabetic condition had progressed beyond the point where it could be managed by diet and lifestyle and prescribed the standard prescription oral drug Metformin to help control his glucose level. However, the drug made him nauseous, and he stopped taking it. The doctor then prescribed regular insulin injections to stabilize his condition.

Like many people who had never had to deal with illness, Gary was frustrated and depressed by this rapid deterioration of his condition. How could he have developed a diabetic condition that required insulin shots so quickly, especially after he followed the doctor's advice? He shared his frustration with his daughter, who suggested that he get a second opinion. At first, Gary was reluctant to get involved with more doctors but after thinking about having to inject himself with insulin for the rest of his life—he agreed. She suggested the doctor whom she was seeing who specialized in a more holistic, natural approach to health issues and was certified in AK. Skeptical but willing to try a different approach, he made an appointment.

At the doctor's office, Gary completed the patient profile, and, during the consultation, the doctor quickly learned several important facts. Gary was a recovering alcoholic. He always had a craving for sweets and carbohydrate type foods (bread, pasta, and especially pancakes). He drank only coffee and iced tea, both sweetened with four packets of sugar, and rarely drank water.

The doctor also noted that Gary had distinct white spots on several of his fingernails which indicated a condition known as leukonychia. This condition is often associated with a zinc deficiency. Zinc is one of the elements vital to the production, storage, and action of natural insulin. A zinc deficiency can predispose a person to diabetes.

Both Postural and Gait Analysis revealed a pronounced elevation of Gary's left shoulder. This postural pattern is associated with a dysfunction of the latissimus dorsi (lat) muscle, which could account for his shoulder pain. This muscle also has been observed to have a strong correlation to blood sugar disturbances and pancreatic function.

During the physical examination, functional muscle testing of the patient's shoulder confirmed inhibition of the left latissimus dorsi muscle. Then the doctor had Gary Therapy Localize by putting light pressure on the left side of his ribcage between the seventh and eighth ribs with his right hand, where the neurolymphatic (NL) skin receptors for the pancreas are located. The muscle became physiologically stronger when the muscle was tested again—indicating a neural "misfiring" of these mechanoreceptors. The interruption of these signals can cause muscle dysfunction and affect the nearby pancreas gland.

Next, the doctor had Gary perform a taste test for zinc. This simple test is performed by having the patient swish around a 0.1% zinc sulfate solution in his mouth for ten seconds and tell the doctor immediately what it tastes like. If successful, the patient would note some kind of mineral/metallic taste. If not, he would not be able to taste much of anything at all. Gary failed to taste the zinc, which indicated that he had a serious zinc deficiency.

After reviewing his blood tests, the doctor concluded that Gary was suffering from a dysfunction of the pancreas, which may or may not have been full-blown diabetes. The pain in his shoulder indicated that there was some kind of problem with the *latissimus dorsi* (lat) muscle, which is the broadest muscle in the body. Muscles can play a significant role in the regulation of blood sugar levels, because they work with insulin to draw in glucose from the blood, thus lowering blood sugar levels. Therapeutically, an optimally functioning large muscle like the *lat* can be a big help in this regard. In this case, treatment of the mechanoreceptors between the ribs could free up any intercostal (ribcage) restrictions and any inhibition of neural signals to the *lat* muscle and, by association, the pancreas—in an attempt to help normalize blood sugar levels.

Mechanical corrections can normalize this neural input to the pancreas and, along with zinc supplementation, can physiologically restore normal function to the pancreas, enabling it to produce enough insulin to balance an individual's glucose levels naturally. If the treatments were successful, insulin injections might not be necessary.

The doctor began Gary's treatment by vigorously stimulating NL skin mechanoreceptors for 30 seconds, after which Gary remarked that his shoulder pain had decreased. The Applied Kinesiologist taught Gary how to stimulate these reflexes at home for thirty seconds daily to provide therapeutic stimulation to the shoulder muscle and the related organ: his pancreas. He was instructed to do this for one month.

The Applied Kinesiologist proceeded to put Gary on a high-quality zinc supplement and recommended that he introduce foods high in zinc into his diet including oysters, grass-fed beef, lamb, chicken, spinach, cashews, mushrooms and, especially, raw pumpkin seeds. To curb his craving for sweets, the doctor also recommended a liquid solution of the herb *gymnema sylestre*. Not only has *gymnema* been shown to lower blood glucose levels, but it also alters the taste sensation of sweetness so that if the patient takes a bite of something sweet, it actually tastes almost like cardboard.

The doctor also suggested that Gary increase his physical activity with daily isometric exercises and pushups, which burn excess glucose effectively and continue with the long walks prescribed by the medical doctor. Finally, he had Gary drink 64 oz of water daily and cut back on his bread, pasta, pancakes, and most especially, his sweet coffee and tea consumption. The doctor suggested he flavor the hot coffee with ½ a teaspoon of olive or coconut oil instead, and to drink his iced tea plain. Gary balked but agreed to try it.

Gary saw the Applied Kinesiologist weekly for two months. The treatments focused on improving physiological function of the large *latissimus* muscle along with various modalities to help optimize blood sugar balance including muscle facilitation, spinal manipulations and stimulating acupuncture points. To check his progress, he used his home glucose monitor and checked his levels regularly. After the first two months of AK treatments, isometric exercises, and taking zinc and *gymnema sylestre*, his blood glucose levels fluctuated between 99 and 120. By month four, they had settled at under 100—a normal reading.

His new diet and exercise regimen helped him lose fourteen additional pounds. As his zinc levels became normal, he switched from a zinc supplement to a multi-mineral one to ensure getting the required amount of zinc, copper, manganese, chromium, and other minerals essential for proper blood sugar metabolism and good health in general. Gary had his sweet cravings under control, so he stopped taking the *gymnema sylestre*. He experienced no shoulder pain, his urinary frequency was vastly improved (even with the increased water consumption), and he no longer had the white spots on his fingernails. He also related that he had grown to prefer the smooth taste of the oil in his coffee as well as drinking his iced tea without sugar.

Gary went back to his medical doctor and had the same battery of blood tests to check his condition. They confirmed that he no longer had any signs of Type 2 diabetes. Gary continues to stay active, do his exercises, keep to his diet (with the occasional pancake breakfast), and enjoy his retirement.

HYPOTHYROIDISM

The thyroid gland is a butterfly-shaped organ that sits in the front of your neck. It has a significant role in regulating many aspects of our metabolism, including breathing, heart rate, blood pressure, body weight and temperature, muscle strength, cholesterol levels, and menstrual cycles, through its production of the hormones T3 (triiodothyronine) and T4 (thyroxine). It uses specific nutrients such as iodine, selenium, protein and vitamin B6 from the foods you eat to make these hormones.

The thyroid is enveloped by thyro-laryngeal fascia, a visceral fascia that is part of the deep cervical fascia of your neck called the pretracheal fascial layer. Underneath this fascial covering, your thyroid has another thin covering that encapsulates the gland and extends into the gland itself, where it divides it into various compartments called lobes and lobules. A layer of thyroid cartilage commonly known as the Adam's apple sits above the thyroid and protects your vocal cords.

Principal neural control of the thyroid gland comes from the autonomic nervous system. Parasympathetic fibers are associated with the vagus nerve, and sympathetic fibers are distributed from the superior, middle, and inferior cervical ganglia of the sympathetic trunk. These small nerves enter the gland along with blood vessels. The parasympathetic fibers have a calming effect on your nervous system and, along with the vagus nerve, stimulate the release of digestive enzymes and hormones. The sympathetic fibers are linked to the stress response, which causes the release of hormones that increase the body's metabolism and energy distribution.

The hypothalamus gland, a tiny structure located inside the brain and attached to the pituitary gland, regulates the thyroid gland. It produces the hormone TRH (thyrotropin-releasing hormone) that tells the pituitary gland to secrete the hormone TSH (thyroid-stimulating hormone) which, in turn, governs the thyroid. Any interruption in the production of either of these hormones can result in a dysfunction of the thyroid.

Hypothyroidism is a condition in which the thyroid is not producing enough hormones. Symptoms of hypothyroidism include fatigue, weight gain, increased sensitivity to cold, constipation, dry skin, throat hoarseness, difficulty swallowing, irregular menstrual periods, muscular weakness, depression, hair loss, high cholesterol, and trouble remembering things.

Hyperthyroidism is the opposite, wherein the gland is producing too many hormones. Symptoms of hyperthyroidism include rapid heartbeat, an enlarged thyroid, nervousness, anxiety, sweating, increased sensitivity to heat, sudden weight loss, difficulty sleeping, brittle hair, and menstrual irregularities. Either condition can cause serious health problems.

An estimated 200 million people in the world suffer from some kind of thyroid problem.[37] The American Thyroid Association states that an estimated 20 million Americans have some form of thyroid disease with up to 60% unaware of their condition.[38]

* * *

GAIL, 33, was a dynamic literary agent who was a master at multitasking, juggling projects, and arranging meetings to the amazement of her colleagues. However, over a period of a few months, her intense energy seemed to be slipping away. She started to gain weight, despite her vigorous gym schedule and attention to her strict vegan diet. Her skin lost its elasticity, and she was constantly cold. She would suddenly start crying for no apparent reason and suffered from depression. Gradually, it got to the point where she no longer recognized herself—physically and emotionally.

She went to her medical doctor, who immediately knew something was off with her endocrine system as she explained the symptoms. Blood tests displayed a high level of TSH and low levels of both T3 and T4, suggesting that Gail was suffering from hypothyroidism. He prescribed thyroxine, a synthetic thyroid hormone to help balance the effects of her condition. She was elated to have a simple diagnosis with a simple "cure." She began taking this supplemental hormone and soon felt like her old energetic self within a few days.

Her elation was short-lived, however. Instead of feeling positive and energetic, she soon became irritable and hyperactive. After two weeks on the medication, she woke up in the middle of the night with heart palpitations, profuse sweating, and hand trembling—and had to go to the emergency room. The ER tests showed that her heart was fine, but now her blood tests exhibited elevated thyroid hormones. These elevated hormone levels, along with the heart palpitations, sweats, irritability, and overall nervousness, were classic signs of *hyper*thyroidism. The emergency room personnel suggested that she consult with her physician to lower her prescribed dosage of thyroxine. Gail complied, and her doctor decreased her dosage. But once again, within a few weeks, she soon complained that her original lethargy returned. The doctor referred her to an endocrinologist for further evaluation.

The endocrinologist palpated her thyroid and said that it felt somewhat swollen. He ordered more in-depth blood tests and found elevated thyroid peroxidase antibody levels, which indicates an autoimmune disease known as Hashimoto's thyroiditis.

Hashimoto's thyroiditis is the most common cause of hypothyroidism in the United States. It occurs when the antibodies of your immune system mistakenly attack the thyroid gland causing swelling and gradual destruction of the gland. When this occurs, eventually the thyroid is unable to make its hormones. There is no medical cure for this condition.

The doctor suggested that she could add the T3 hormone to the thyroxine and see how that goes. Gail agreed to try it. Once again, she felt better initially, then relapsed. Her specialist said that the next step would involve removing the thyroid gland, either by surgery or radiation, and putting her on permanent hormone replacement. She was so miserable that she said she would seriously consider these radical measures but first wanted to get a second opinion.

Gail researched her condition and discovered a wide range of alternative methods of treatment. She found a holistic doctor specializing in AK who, according to testimonials from patients with similar conditions, had success in curing people suffering from hypothyroidism through non-drug related or non-invasive treatments. She made an appointment.

During her initial consultation, the doctor reviewed her medical records and seemed to support the diagnosis of Hashimoto's Thyroiditis. However, he also felt that the specialist was being a little aggressive in so quickly suggesting hormone replacement therapy and the additional suggestion that the removal of her thyroid might be necessary.

He explained that many factors might contribute to her condition; one major factor being diet. Gail shared that a few years ago before she started having problems, she had adopted a strict vegan diet and began drinking copious amounts of green tea during the day from her local coffee shop. The doctor informed her that people who adopted a strict vegan diet often suffered from a lack of B6, B12, iodine, and selenium—all vital for proper thyroid function. He then asked if she drank her tea from disposal coffee shop cups with plastic lids. Surprised at the question, she said she did. He shared with her that those disposable lids contained high levels of BPA (Bisphenol A), an endocrine disrupting chemical that inhibits thyroid function.

Postural Analysis displayed that Gail stood with her palms facing directly behind her instead of facing her sides. This is a common posture for people suffering from hypothyroidism. This occurs because of the relationship of the thyroid to the teres *minor*, the shoulder muscle that rotates the arm outwards. When there is thyroid dysfunction, the compromised muscle will cause the hands to turn in, and the knuckles will face forward. This muscle imbalance can lead to shoulder problems as well, a common complaint in people with hypothyroidism.[39] Gait Analysis showed the same "knuckles forward" position when she walked.

The doctor began his physical examination by palpating the thyroid and the surrounding area in the front of the throat and noted that it was slightly swollen but not to the extent that is usual in Hashimoto's Thyroiditis. He went further to feel the scalene and hyoid muscles on the sides and front of the neck, respectively. Gail winced; her muscles were abnormally tight causing her pain when touched. Next, he asked if her exercise routine included sit-ups, using the traditional hands-behind-the neck position. She replied that it did. He also asked if she put any other stress on her neck; she explained that she regularly read in bed with her head propped forward on her pillow.

The doctor reached for a 128 Hz tuning fork, struck it on the examination table to induce vibration, and placed it over several areas on the front of her neck, then tested her muscles. The Vibration Challenge resulted in a physiological muscle weakness. The same phenomenon occurred when the vibrating tuning fork was placed over the breastbone in front of the thymus gland. These findings indicated a thickening of the fascia underlying the vibrating tuning fork. Further investigation revealed that the sixth cervical vertebra in the back of the neck was misaligned.

The doctor shared his initial diagnosis of the factors that contributed to the patient's condition. Her blood tests revealed that Gail had a B12, iodine, and possible protein deficiency—commonly found in people avoiding all animal products. These deficiencies did not give her thyroid gland the necessary substances for it to produce sufficient quantities of the hormones she needed.

More importantly, the constant stresses on her neck from reading in bed and sit-ups had tightened the fascia of her neck and upper chest causing a subluxation of her neck bone, which interrupted the normal nerve impulses to the thyroid gland. Additionally, the sternothyroid muscle that covers the lateral surface of the thyroid and connects to the breastbone (sternum) was in spasm due to a thickening in its fascia and, along with the tightened thyroid fascia, was "strangling" her thyroid.

The Applied Kinesiologist asserted that these fascial restrictions could be impacting the lymphatic drainage of the thyroid gland and result in the congestion or "swelling" of the area. The specialist's initial diagnosis of Hashimoto's Thyroiditis was based on the blood test and the slight swelling of the thyroid. In Gail's case, the lymphatic drainage appeared to be a significant contributor to her symptoms; this appeared to be a clear reason for her *lymphocytes* attacking her thyroid, potentially leading to her auto-immune imbalance.

Applied Kinesiologists often find that "autoimmune problems" are secondary manifestations of dysfunction of either the adrenal glands or the thymus gland. The thymus gland is the main regulator of the lymphatic system. It is located behind your breastbone at the level of your heart and is covered by thick connective tissue. The thymus gland stores immune cells called T (thymus) cells. T cells are *lymphocytes* formed in your bone marrow that travel to your thymus gland until they mature enough to fulfill their role in identifying and attacking intruding foreign bodies (antigens) in the body. If the T cells are released prematurely, they can mistakenly attack parts of the body they are designed to protect—including the thyroid.

The doctor explained that since her thyroid gland was not functioning because of the pressure from its surrounding fascia, it became inflamed. The thymus, which also appeared to be dysfunctional due to its own fascial constriction, released a high level of immature T cells that attacked the thyroid, leading to elevated levels of thyroid peroxidase associated with Hashimoto's Thyroiditis.

Gail responded that this sounded far-fetched, especially the physical constriction of the muscles and fascia affecting the glands. She thought that it was strictly a matter of a hormone imbalance caused by the dysfunction of her thyroid gland. The doctor agreed, but the underlying cause of the thyroid dysfunction was the constriction of her thyroid by the surrounding muscles and fascia, not a fundamental problem with the gland itself. He suggested that once this tension was relieved, it would allow her thyroid to begin to function more normally and eliminate the swelling. Subsequent treatment to her thymus gland could stop the T cell invasion; thus, relieving the autoimmune component of her problem. Together with attention to her diet, exercise and reading habits, her condition could be greatly improved or cured; without further juggling of synthetic hormones, surgery, or radiation. Not fully convinced, she hesitantly agreed to try the doctor's suggested course of therapy.

Treatment began with percussion therapy to loosen the pretracheal fascia covering the thyroid, the sternohyoid muscles, and the fascial covering of the sternum, ribs and the thymus gland. Then the doctor applied a precise chiropractic adjustment to restore normal motion to the misaligned bone in Gail's neck to allow healthy nerve function.

The doctor instructed Gail to take nutritional supplements including an easily absorbable form of vitamins B6 and B12 daily for as long as she was avoiding meat; as well as a balanced multimineral capsule that included iodine, selenium, magnesium, zinc, copper, manganese, and molybdenum, to ensure that she had the other minerals essential to good thyroid health. He suggested that she also take the herbs *astragalus* and *maitake* to support the thymus gland. This would help her in developing mature T Cells to correct the "autoimmune" aspect of her problem.

The Applied Kinesiologist also referred Gail to a nutritionist to educate her on a more balanced approach to her vegan diet, as well as include the nutrients she was lacking that are necessary for proper thyroid function. The doctor gave her advice about healthier abdominal exercises and reading positions to prevent stress on her neck. Finally, he advised her to stop drinking out of cups with disposable plastic lids.

Gail felt the benefits of the treatment over the following week. Her energy returned, and her mood was considerably better. She required weekly treatments for two months and then once a month over the next year. During this time, she dropped the twenty pounds that she had gained. Her thyroid levels are all in the normal range, and her autoimmune condition has disappeared.

* * *

Hormones are vital to the proper functioning of your body. Any hormone imbalance can create serious health problems. Traditional medicine often treats many hormone conditions, such as diabetes and hypothyroidism, by using synthetic substitutes to restore balance to hormone levels. It is a dangerous game and can take months to adjust the levels properly, while the patient suffers the effects. If this treatment proves unsuccessful, the next step in traditional medicine to attempt hormonal equilibrium may be more drugs to suppress your immune system, insulin pumps, or gland removal with surgery or destruction with radiation.

Applied Kinesiology takes another approach. AK doctors employ noninvasive techniques, including functional muscle testing, to reveal the physical source of the dysfunction and correct it by using receptor-based therapies—such as chiropractic adjustments and AK techniques—to restore the proper function of the glands. Supported by precise attention to the nutritional needs of glands and lifestyle choices, this approach can address most nonpathological hormonal conditions.

13
RESPIRATORY CONDITIONS

Breathing is the single most important activity in our lives. We inhale and exhale approximately 20,000 times[40] and process about 11,000 liters[41] of air daily. We take in oxygen with every breath which is necessary for our body to function and expel carbon dioxide, a waste byproduct which is poisonous in high concentrations. While our lungs are the principal organ responsible for gathering and processing the air we breathe, they are dependent upon the movement of the diaphragm and ribcage and, to a lesser degree, the abdominal muscles and connecting spinal joints, to allow us to breathe in and out. The dynamic functioning of this system represents the critical components of healthy respiration.

When you breathe in, your diaphragm flattens; pushing out the lower ribs and stomach and expanding the chest cavity. This downward motion draws air in through your nose and/or mouth down the trachea (windpipe) and through your vocal cords in the larynx until it reaches the bronchi. Air then passes into your right and left lungs and continues through the bronchioles until it enters air sacs called alveoli. Your lungs have about 480,000,000 alveoli,[42] and the oxygen you inhale enters these air sacs where it passes into the capillaries and into the bloodstream. As oxygen is going into the bloodstream, carbon dioxide passes from the blood into the alveoli and out of the body with expiration.

When you breathe out, the diaphragm relaxes and moves upward bringing the intercostal muscles between your ribs closer together to reduce the size of the chest cavity. Along with the elastic lung tissue, this reduction in space helps to push the carbon dioxide and excess air up through the trachea and out through the nostrils and mouth. When you need to expel carbon dioxide quickly, such as during exercise, the abdominal muscles contract to accelerate the expiration process as well.

Various factors can affect the health of your lungs and breathing system such as genetic disposition, smoking, poor diet, dehydration, infections, allergens, and serious pathological conditions. Some of those conditions include asthma, tuberculosis, emphysema, pneumonia, bronchitis, lung infections, chronic obstructive pulmonary disease (COPD), and lung cancer.

Applied Kinesiologists can help diagnose and cure people of many lung conditions caused by or made worse by dysfunction in the total breathing mechanism. Additionally, AK therapies can ensure proper maintenance of the neural connections that control your respiratory muscles as well as other bodily systems not commonly thought of as supporting healthy lung function.

ASTHMA

Asthma is a chronic lung disease that inflames and constricts your airways. Symptoms include episodes of wheezing, chest tightness, coughing, and shortness of breath. The most recent estimate suggests that 334,000,000 people worldwide have asthma,[43] including 25,000,000 Americans[44] with 7,000,000 of those being children.[44]

Asthma attacks generally coincide with stressors such as physical exertion, anxiety, breathing cold, dry air, or allergies. Irritants in the air, including smoke, chemical fumes and strong odors such as perfumes, can also trigger attacks. Your genetic makeup can predispose you to develop asthma, which is why asthma generally starts in childhood. The Center for Disease Control (CDC) reports that a person who has a parent that has asthma is up to 6 times as likely to develop asthma than someone who does not have a parent with asthma.[45] While many children with asthma experience lessening symptoms as they reach adulthood, they tend to remain susceptible to attacks—usually under times of duress, anxiety or strong physical exertion.

While traditional medicine views asthma as a condition centered in the lungs themselves, Applied Kinesiologists, along with other functional medicine specialists, have found asthma to be less of a lung problem and more of a dysfunction of the systems essential to proper lung function, especially during times of duress. One of your body's first responses to stimuli, such as emotional stress, physical exertion, pollutants, or an allergen is a dilation of your airways to accommodate more oxygen, which sets in motion the rest of the body's breathing system. This response is regulated in large part by your adrenal glands and the autonomic nervous system.

Essentially, your autonomic nervous system consists of two complementary systems: the parasympathetic system which maintains such routine functions as breathing, digestion, and sleep, and the sympathetic system which alerts the body to respond to stressful situations. Your adrenal glands modulate the proper response of your sympathetic nervous system to ensure that your lungs supply you with the necessary oxygen during those times of increased demand by producing hormones that dilate the airways.

The parasympathetic nervous system releases the neurotransmitter *acetylcholine* which causes the natural constriction of the smooth muscle layer surrounding the bronchi. The sympathetic nervous system releases the hormone *epinephrine* to *relax* the smooth muscles lining the bronchi, resulting in dilation of the airways and an increase of your supply of oxygen. When there is an imbalance in these two systems, bronchial spasms can occur in times of stress—whether emotional or physiological. The most common cause of this imbalance is adrenal fatigue. When the adrenal glands are not secreting enough hormones (adrenaline and cortisol), your airways constrict instead of dilating in times of stress or exertion. This leads to the *gasping for air* symptom seen in asthma attacks.

AK treatments restore equilibrium to the parasympathetic and the sympathetic aspects of your autonomic nervous system to maintain the proper neural impulses to your breathing apparatus. Treatments vary with each individual. The most common and effective therapies successfully address the underlying Adrenal Fatigue Syndrome (AFS), as well as your respiratory mechanism, includes the mobilization of the ribcage, the diaphragm, and the cranial bones surrounding the respiratory control center in the brainstem. Once the underlying imbalance in your nervous system is *recalibrated*, the inappropriate stress response is normalized, and the asthma symptoms can be permanently eradicated.

While it is obvious to most people that improving the respiratory mechanism can help with breathing difficulties; it is not as obvious that adrenal fatigue plays a major role in asthma. Applied Kinesiologists have empirically found that AFS is a major contributor to the symptoms found in asthmatic patients. This helps to explain why the two most common medications prescribed for people suffering from asthma are *corticosteroids* and others that mimic or contain adrenaline or *epinephrine*—drugs based upon hormones naturally secreted by your *adrenal glands*. These medications are used to decrease inflammation, relieve constriction, and dilate the bronchioles by relaxing the tightened muscles around your airways.

* * *

STEVE, 32, had suffered from asthma his entire life. His parents were divorcing while his mother was pregnant with him. Some studies have shown that if a mother is under chronic stress during pregnancy, adrenal hormones are released into the amniotic fluid. Children of these mothers are prone to have health issues such as asthma, allergies, respiratory illness, behavioral problems, and premature delivery. At the age of ten, he started to experience severe shortness of breath when he became anxious and when playing basketball; by twelve years old, it had worsened to the point where he could no longer play baseball, even with an inhaler in the back pocket of his uniform.

He was relegated from sports participant to spectator at a young age because of his asthma attacks. But he loved sports, and despite his inability to play, he eventually pursued his dream career as a successful sportswriter. As long as he stayed away from physical exertion and excessively stressful situations, his asthma remained under control.

The birth of his first son brought him a deep feeling of joy, as well as many sleepless nights due to the baby's colic. This loss of his usual sound sleep impacted his system and brought back his asthma attacks with a vengeance. He had not experienced these attacks in years; they caught him completely off guard. Even his simple exercise program of bike riding now triggered his asthma. He went to see his longtime family doctor who knew his medical history and prescribed an inhaler; he had not used one for years. After using it, he experienced headaches, dizziness, and overall nervousness and tremors.

Finding his reaction to the inhaler odd, his medical doctor referred him to a pulmonary specialist, who confirmed the diagnosis of asthma and switched Steve to yet another inhaler. When Steve again suffered from headaches along with new symptoms of dry mouth and throat hoarseness, the doctor prescribed Steve an oral steroid (prednisone) to try to get the symptoms under control, prevent the attacks, and limit the use of the inhalers. Steve balked at taking the steroid pill when he read about the long-term side effects of using corticosteroids—meanwhile, his attacks and other symptoms continued. The source of the resurgence of these attacks remained unclear.

At this time, Steve's wife spoke to another parent at a Mommy and Me class about her son's colic. The mother mentioned that an Applied Kinesiologist had helped her daughter who suffered with it. Steve and his wife made an appointment with their son. While at the doctor's office, Steve noticed some literature in the reception room about natural help for people suffering from breathing problems such as asthma. When his son's treatment was done, Steve asked the doctor about his asthma. The doctor said that he had good success in helping people with it. Steve made an appointment for himself the following week.

During the initial consultation, Steve shared that he had suffered from asthma all his life. He had always been able to control it with inhalers, but they didn't seem to be working anymore. He hadn't had a serious attack until his son was born and his usual sleep patterns had become interrupted. When the doctor inquired about his diet, Steve said he was a "meat and potatoes" person and rarely ate vegetables or fruit. Due to his asthma, he didn't do any strenuous exercise and limited his activity to bicycling.

Postural Analysis showed that Steve tended to slouch when he stood. Slouching creates a continual cycle of stress to the muscles in the rib cage and affects its ability to expand enough for the lungs to operate normally. Gait Analysis revealed the same slumping posture, as well as the additional observation that Steve had no "bounce" at all to his step. In fact, he walked so lethargically that it looked like he was walking in *slow motion*.

The doctor began the physical examination by testing the calf muscles that are responsible for propelling you forward when you walk. Functional muscle testing revealed a distinct physiological inhibition of both gastrocnemius (calf) muscles. In AK, a non-traumatic (not due to an injury) inhibition of the calf muscles often points to an apparent dysfunction of the muscles and fascia closely linked to the adrenal glands. Further evaluation revealed that his rib cage was restricted when he breathed.

The doctor tested his blood pressure while sitting and again when standing. Steve's blood pressure dropped when he went from sitting to standing, and the doctor noted that his pupils could not retain their constriction when a penlight shined in them for ten seconds. Both these responses were signs of imbalance in his system. The doctor proceeded to have Steve blow into a small machine called a spirometer. This medical device measures the amount of air you breathe out and the speed of your breath. The normal spirometer reading for a healthy thirty-two-year-old man is approximately 4000 c.c. Steve's ventilation numbers were 2800 c.c., which means he had severely limited lung capacity even when he was breathing normally.

The doctor had Steve perform a taste test with licorice and noticed an immediate positive reaction. The root of *Glycyrrhiza glabra,* commonly known as licorice, has been shown to increase the efficacy of adrenal steroids in the body and is a potent stimulant in helping your adrenal medulla make catecholamines, such as adrenaline. It also helps restore function to the gastrocnemius muscles on both sides, stabilizes blood pressure, and relieves the loss of pupillary constriction to light—all linked to adrenal hormone deficiency.

All this information pointed to a general dysfunction in Steve's entire breathing system, excluding his lungs. The doctor concluded that the patient's asthma was the result of ongoing stress caused by his sleep deprivation. Sleep is proven to be critical to the normal functioning of your central nervous system, and this loss of restorative sleep caused his adrenal glands to work overtime to produce adrenal medulla and cortical hormones that help cope with the stress. Since the stress of sleep loss was continual, the adrenals could not keep up, and Steve developed Adrenal Fatigue Syndrome (AFS). The condition had become so severe that even when Steve returned to a normal sleeping pattern after the doctor relieved his son's colic, his system would remain compromised unless treated.

The doctor explained to Steve that inhalers commonly given to asthma sufferers to facilitate breathing during an asthma attack deliver a quick dose of adrenal hormones directly to the bronchia in the lungs. In his case, the AFS was so progressed that the inhalers were unable to make up for the hormone deficiency. Not only were they not as effective, but they produced Steve's other symptoms not usually associated with asthma.

The doctor said they would need to treat the AFS to reset his body's hormonal balance and relieve the current symptoms. As part of the treatment, they would address his diet and stress management as well. Steve was a bit hesitant, as neither his family doctor nor the pulmonary specialist had ever mentioned AFS as being linked to his asthma. The AK specialist said that it was difficult for traditional medical doctors to detect AFS and often assigned its symptoms to other conditions. The doctor reiterated that since adrenal hormones are the medications given to help people suffering from asthma, it makes sense that asthma must be a secondary condition to the underlying adrenal problem. Steve agreed to try this approach.

First, the doctor worked on the dysfunction in the fascial covering of the adrenal glands to relieve the stress on the glands. The constriction of this fascial covering also affected the most important of the respiratory muscles—the diaphragm. A fascial restriction could affect its primary function of supporting the expansion and contraction of the lungs.

Next, the Applied Kinesiologist treated the skin mechanoreceptors over the sternum (breastbone) and between the second, third, and fourth ribs and where the 12th rib connects with the spine in the back. The receptors had become inhibited by Steve's poor posture. With thirty seconds of vigorous stimulation, these receptors relaxed the muscles surrounding the ribcage. Restoring both the function of these receptors and the fascia in turn facilitated the normal adrenals to release *epinephrine* (adrenaline) which *relaxed* the smooth muscles lining the bronchi and opened up the airways.

The doctor then applied precise adjustive therapy to enable full movement of the chest muscles, thoracic spine, and ribs. Steve had never experienced chiropractic adjustments before and was amazed at the freedom of movement he now experienced in his ribcage, spine, and even his shoulders. He raised his arms up and outwards and told the doctor that he just took the deepest breath he could ever remember.

Steve came in for biweekly visits for two weeks, weekly visits for two months, and then monthly visits for 6 months. After two months, his spirometer readings improved to 3800 c.c. which were more in line with his optimal breathing levels. During this period, the doctor recommended that Steve take licorice root once a day between 9:00 a.m. and 11:00 a.m.—the time that the adrenal glands secrete maximal levels of the stress hormone cortisol. Cortisol is important for many reasons, one of them being its critical function as a powerful anti-inflammatory, especially for the bronchi in the lungs. This can help relieve any possible restriction in your airways due to inflammation.

The Applied Kinesiologist recommended that Steve start taking a vitamin C complex with bioflavonoids and begin including more vegetables and fruits in his diet. The doctor showed him a calming, deep breathing, rib-opening exercise for him to perform six times a day to help keep the spine and ribcage straight and supple as well as postural exercises to help him break the slouching habit. He suggested that Steve walk thirty minutes a day whenever possible, as mild exercise supports good health but will not trigger any respiratory problems and will keep his spine and ribs upright and open.

After the first month, nearly all of Steve's symptoms had disappeared. He then switched from licorice root to a more general adrenal tonic—Panax ginseng herbal supplement—that he takes daily. Along with being an adaptogen to help balance Steve's nervous system, Panax ginseng has been found in studies to reverse lung damage caused by asthma over the years. He adjusted his diet to include more vegetables and fruits and kept to his mild exercise routine. His asthma disappeared.

Vocal Cord Dysfunction Syndrome

Vocal cord dysfunction (VCD), also called laryngeal dysfunction, is the abnormal closing of the vocal cords. It makes breathing difficult and is often mistaken for asthma. It can be triggered by inhaling lung irritants such as tobacco smoke, upper respiratory infections, or extreme physical activity. Symptoms of VCD include a sensation of tightness in the throat or chest, shortness of breath and difficulty getting air into or out of your lungs, a feeling of choking or suffocation, the need to frequently cough or clear your throat, noisy breathing, and the development of a hoarse or raspy voice. The usual medical treatments to address these symptoms include special breathing exercises involving panting maneuvers, along with psycho-therapeutic behavioral and speech therapies.

* * *

SALLY, 16, was an excellent high school lacrosse player. She loved the sport and the camaraderie with her best friends who were all on the team. After having suffered from an upper respiratory infection, she found herself gasping for breath at lacrosse practice. It frightened her and her teammates, as well as her parents. The family doctor could not find any cause for her condition. The best diagnosis she could give was that it was some kind of asthmatic condition; she advised Sally to use an inhaler whenever it happened. She and her parents were surprised, as they had no history of asthma in the family, and Sally had never experienced problems with breathing before. The doctor also told Sally that it would be wise to give up lacrosse until a definitive diagnosis could be made. She recommended a pulmonologist.

The pulmonary specialist ran several breathing tests and found nothing wrong with her lungs. When he put her on the treadmill, she was also fine. The doctor then had her do jumping jacks; after one minute, she was gasping for breath and felt constriction in her throat. He had cervical X-rays and an MRI done, but everything seemed normal. The doctor was stumped and suggested that they consult with an otolaryngologist or throat specialist.

The specialist examined Sally's throat and trachea and didn't see any pathological problems. She had no problem swallowing or breathing normally. He theorized that physical exertion might be impacting her throat muscles, causing what appeared to be VCD syndrome. He suggested that she might benefit from seeing a licensed massage therapist (LMT) to try to relieve any tension in the throat muscles. However, until her symptoms cleared up, he also suggested that she stop playing sports altogether. At the news, Sally cried all the way home—distraught that she would have to give up lacrosse.

The coach let Sally stay on the team, dress for games, and remain on the bench. While her parents were in the stands during one game, the father of one of Sally's friends asked how she was doing. Her mother said she really missed playing with her team and was frustrated that none of the doctors could find what was causing her condition. Not one of the treatments helped her at all. The friend's father suggested that since her problem seemed to be related to the muscles of her throat, perhaps his wife's chiropractor could help. He was trained in the field of AK, which dealt with muscle conditions. Feeling that they had nothing to lose, her parents took the referral.

After filling out the patient profile forms, the doctor met Sally and her parents in the consultation room. The doctor reviewed the medical records. Sally appeared to be in excellent health except for her breathing problem during exercise.

The Applied Kinesiologist inquired more deeply and asked about the upper respiratory infection that was listed on her patient profile. Sally mentioned that she had experienced a bad upper respiratory infection last winter and missed a week of school and practice. When she was feeling better, she returned to practice and started having the attacks. The doctor asked Sally if she were coughing a lot when she had the infection. Sally said she had coughed constantly during that time. She also related that it was right around the time of her breathing problem that she noticed a little trouble swallowing and some popping in the front of her chest when she stood up.

After noting these important bits of information, the four of them proceeded to the examination room. Postural Analysis quickly showed Sally standing slightly hunched over with her head and shoulders locked in a forward position and her chest sunken in. Gait Analysis accentuated this hunched-over position of her head, shoulders, and chest—to the point where she looked like someone was pressing on her chest as she walked down the hall toward the three of them.

The doctor had Sally lie face up on the examination table and palpated the reflex points on both sides of her skull (known as the Temporal Sphenoidal (TS) line that corresponds with the neck muscles) and found tender nodules on both sides. The doctor tested Sally's front neck flexor muscles and found them severely inhibited. More strikingly, immediately after the test, Sally began to experience the very same throat constriction and difficulty breathing that had been plaguing her on the field. After she was able to breathe normally, he proceeded with the examination.

When the doctor palpated the upper part of the sternum (breastbone), Sally gasped in pain. He once again tested Sally's neck flexor muscles, this time while she held her hand on the painful area of her breastbone and exerted a slight pressure to lift it upward. This improved muscle function dramatically, facilitating her breathing without pain.

The Applied Kinesiologist confirmed the diagnosis of the throat specialist that Sally had VCD. He deduced that her continual deep coughing during her upper respiratory infection had caused the *manubriosternal* joint at the top part of the breastbone to lock into position, resulting in a physiological dysfunction of the delicate muscles in the front of Sally's neck. This would explain why the treadmill test at the pulmonologist did not elicit respiratory distress, but jumping jacks did. When shoulder and ribcage movement was vigorously engaged, such as in jumping jacks or running with a lacrosse stick, the inhibited neck muscles that connect to the collarbone, ribs, and cervical spine could not handle the stress. Consequently, Sally's laryngeal muscles (vocal cords) would go into spasm and restrict the airways. These laryngeal muscles are critical for swallowing, speaking, coughing, and breathing.

The doctor explained that treatment would begin by addressing the jamming of the sternum and the restricted cervical vertebrae. This would facilitate the neural control to the neck flexor muscles and relieve the resultant spasm of the hyoid muscles affecting the trachea or windpipe. Once the proper function of the muscles and alignment of bone structures were restored, her condition should disappear. Sally and her parents, relieved that they finally got a comprehensive diagnosis of Sally's condition, agreed for the doctor to start the treatment plan.

Treatment began immediately to restore normal motion to the bones in the neck. The doctor used an adjusting tool called the Arthostim® and directed several gentle thrusts in a counter-rotation direction on the various fixated cervical vertebrae. The doctor then relieved the tension in the neck and throat muscles through manual manipulation of their spindle cells (the receptors in the muscle that maintain normal muscle tone).

Next, the doctor would need to restore the normal position to the upper sternum. He put a hot pack over the area for ten minutes to loosen up the manubriosternal joint while Sally took long, slow, deep breaths. The doctor then placed his hands at the jammed joint, which is slightly above where you would place your hands if you were giving someone CPR. Instead of pressing straight down on the sternum, the doctor pressed upward to lift the manubrium off the body of the sternum. Immediately, Sally gasped as air rushed into her lungs, unimpeded by the compressed breastbone. The doctor placed a cold pack over the area to prevent any soreness from the procedure.

Sally rested for ten minutes. After removing the cold pack, the Applied Kinesiologist retested Sally's neck flexor muscles and found them working normally. Sally stood up straighter than before and took a deep breath—deeper than she had taken in many weeks.

Since her muscles were now functioning normally, the doctor suggested that she work with a speech therapist to help strengthen her vocal cords with exercises. Sally returned for biweekly treatments over the next month. A final reevaluation showed that she had fully recovered from her VCD syndrome. She said that she felt great and proved her point by doing 25 jumping jacks with no effort. Impressed, the doctor gave her the green light to return to the sport she loved.

BRONCHITIS

Bronchitis is the inflammation of the lining of the bronchial tubes that carry air to and from your lungs. There are two types of bronchitis: acute and chronic. Acute bronchitis is often referred to as a chest cold and generally lasts about a week, although the cough that usually accompanies it may linger for several weeks. It is most often caused by a viral infection.

Chronic bronchitis begins with a deep cough with mucous that persists for at least three months and recurs throughout a patient's lifetime. It is a condition that affects cigarette smokers and people sensitive to air pollution and respiratory allergies. It is one of the conditions included under the category of chronic obstructive pulmonary disease (COPD). Symptoms of both types of bronchitis include a deep cough with mucus, chest discomfort, fatigue, shortness of breath, and slight chills and fever.

The traditional medical treatments for bronchitis are generally focused upon alleviating symptoms. Bed rest is usually recommended. Additionally, doctors will often prescribe medications to open obstructed airways and thin the mucus within the lungs so that the patient can cough up the sputum more readily. In cases of chronic bronchitis, doctors will impress upon the patient the importance of avoiding environmental irritants, most notably cigarette smoke.

* * *

HANS, 66, was a world-renowned chef. He had tremendous energy and passion for his work. Despite his grueling work schedule, he was dedicated to his overall health. He regularly went for chiropractic treatments and massages, exercised, ate sensibly, and was rarely sick. One winter, he developed a lingering cough which developed into what appeared to be a respiratory problem. It sapped his formidable energy, and he found it difficult to breathe, especially in a hot kitchen. He made an appointment with a general practitioner to find out what might be wrong.

The doctor asked him to inhale and exhale deeply as he listened to his lungs. Hans could not breathe deeply. The doctor took X-rays and noticed that his lungs were severely congested. He diagnosed Hans with acute bronchitis and advised him to rest. He also prescribed antibiotics to prevent him from getting any secondary bacterial infection as he waited for the condition to pass. While Hans did take the antibiotics, he did not take the advice to rest. Unfortunately, after two weeks, his breathing did not get any better. He returned to the medical doctor who, after reexamining Hans, found that his bronchitis had disappeared but could not find any reason why he still had breathing problems.

Hans consulted with his doctor of chiropractic. The chiropractor told him that perhaps a colleague trained in AK might be able to get to the root of this enigmatic upper respiratory problem. She also relayed the fact that many respiratory conditions were linked to muscle dysfunction—a specialty of AK.

During the initial consultation, the AK specialist reviewed the records and could see that both the medical doctor and the doctor of chiropractic were very thorough in their examinations. The patient profile and history revealed that Hans ate predominately wild fish, grass-fed beef, organic vegetables, and fruit, and drank healthy amounts of water. He regularly had chiropractic adjustments, did yoga, and meditated. However, he worked sixteen stress-filled hours six days a week at his new restaurant.

The doctor related that he could see why his case was confusing—Hans seemed to be the "healthiest sick person" he had ever seen. Noteworthy was that Hans mentioned on the extensive questionnaire that he had suffered from a mild case of *intestinal cramping* while traveling several weeks before he started experiencing breathing problems and was currently having intermittent bouts of intestinal discomfort. When the doctor asked him about this, Hans attributed this "knot in his gut" to nerves and the ongoing stress of opening his new restaurant.

Postural, Gait and Temporal/Sphenoidal Line Analysis did not reveal much in the way of serious dysfunction. In the examination room, the doctor proceeded to have Hans blow into a spirometer. Spirometer readings revealed Han's ventilation numbers to be 1700 c.c., roughly that of a 9-year-old boy. Then he had Hans lie face up on the examination table as the doctor proceeded to perform Acupuncture Pulse Point Analysis. This diagnostic procedure has been used in China for thousands of years to find blockages in the body's meridian system. In classical Chinese acupuncture, certain energetic pathways or meridians are coupled or paired with various organs or muscle configurations. As strange as this may seem to western doctors, continuing research has validated that these various points and energy pathways have powerful diagnostic and therapeutic value.

In Hans' case, Acupuncture Pulse Point Analysis revealed a disruption at the point related to the lung/large intestine meridian pathway, indicating an imbalance of energy. The doctor used AK functional muscle testing to find that his right deltoid muscle, a muscle that acts as a measure of lung function, was physiologically inhibited. When the doctor asked Hans to gently touch a point located on the wrist, the right deltoid became physiologically stronger, which confirmed the imbalance. This imbalance could lead to the exact symptoms that Hans displayed: shortness of breath, lack of energy, and intestinal problems.

Further investigation through FMT revealed that the fifth lumbar vertebra was subluxated, affecting the acupuncture point of the large intestine located on the spine between the fourth and fifth lumbar vertebrae. This could explain the energy blockage between the large intestine and the lung. Also, the effects of the antibiotics had probably further impacted the proper functioning of the large intestine—resulting in ongoing digestive problems and impaired lung function.

While the medical doctor's initial diagnosis of acute bronchitis might have explained some of his symptoms, they did not reveal the underlying cause of his condition. Hans' enigmatic breathing problems were related to a combination of spinal misalignment and a disruption in the function of his large intestine. The AK doctor explained that the imbalance in the internal environment (microbiome) of Hans' large intestine contributed to the energy blockage in his lung/large intestine connection, which led to a diminished lung function and the physiological inhibition of his right deltoid muscle.

The treatment began by facilitating the function of Hans' deltoid muscle, helping to free up the upper ribcage; followed by a precise spinal manipulation to the fifth lumbar spinal segment, and acupuncture therapy, using a non-invasive, spring-loaded Tei-shin device, to open up the energy blockage between the large intestine and lung. After these initial adjustments—and the resolution of the underlying problem of his large intestine essentially *stealing* energy from his lungs—Hans noted that his breathing was improved.

To support the role of the large intestine in the healing process, the doctor suggested that Hans take probiotic supplements twice a day for four months. Probiotics are supplements that contain the bacteria necessary for healthy functioning of the intestinal tract. Often, toxins or antibiotics kill this "good" bacteria and affect the natural balance of the immune system. Probiotic supplements were necessary to restore these good bacteria as quickly as possible.

Hans came in for biweekly visits for three weeks. His breathing and energy levels were back to normal with spirometer readings now registering at 4100 c.c., that of a healthy thirty-year-old male, and he no longer had the vague feeling of *tension in his gut*. Functional muscle testing revealed no imbalance in his acupuncture meridian system. He continued to get regular chiropractic adjustments and maintained his diet and exercise regimen. He opened his new restaurant to critical acclaim, and he had no further breathing problems.

* * *

Respiratory problems can be unnerving and a source of tremendous anxiety—the feeling of suffocating while living in a sea of air is terrifying. Unless they are caused by specific pathology, most conditions that impact the complex breathing mechanisms in the body can be traced to a physiological dysfunction in one of these several systems. Through the use of FMT, chiropractic, acupuncture, and muscle manipulation, in conjunction with good nutritional therapy and specific deep breathing exercises, an AK specialist can help the body correct the functional disorders that may be impeding your full respiratory health without the use of pharmaceuticals.

14
HEADACHE DISORDERS

According to the World Health Organization, recurrent headaches, are among the most common disorders of the nervous system. Globally, it is estimated that 50% of adults currently suffer from at least one episode of headache disorders per year.[46] There are two levels of headache disorders: primary and secondary. The majority of primary headache orders are severe and fall into four major categories: migraine, tension-type (TTH), medication-overuse, and cluster headaches. Secondary headaches can range from mild to painful and are usually associated with such physical conditions including sinus infections, eye strain, hypertension, digestive problems, dehydration, and concussions.

According to traditional medicine, primary headaches are caused by overstimulation of the blood vessels, muscles, and nerves of the head and neck leading to increased pressure inside the head. They may also result from changes in chemical activity in the brain due to overmedication or a pathological structure such as a tumor. Since secondary headaches usually arise as a consequence of another condition, traditional medicine tends to treat the condition which, in turn, will relieve the headache. However, if the underlying problem is not diagnosed properly and corrected, the headaches will return.

Applied Kinesiologists believe that the principal nonpathological cause of most headaches can be traced to an imbalance in the expansion and contraction of the bones that make up the skull, which can create a buildup of pressure in your head (*idiopathic intracranial hypertension).* Especially important is the junction between the temporal and occipital cranial bones. The vagus nerve, the longest of the cranial nerves, passes through a space between these bones called the jugular foramen. If this space becomes too narrow due to cranial bone restriction and muscular hypertonicity (tightness), it can impinge upon this nerve—which research has suggested regulates pressure inside the skull and results in headache pain.

Because of its unique approach, AK is particularly well-suited to diagnose and treat the biomechanical and physiological causes of headache disorders. Applied Kinesiologists generally have strong success in curing people of this condition through therapy that restores the proper movement of the cranial bones and nerve function that can cause chronic headaches.

MIGRAINES

Migraine headaches are an enormous problem, affecting more than 1 billion people worldwide,[47] including more than 40 million Americans.[48] Migraines usually begin after the age of 18 and afflict people during their peak productive years, between the ages of 25 and 55 years. It is unclear why migraines affect older adults less frequently. There is no known medical cure for this condition as well.

Migraines typically progress through four stages: prodrome, aura, the actual headache attack, and post-drome. They are:

1. The prodrome stage includes subtle symptoms that occur a day or two before the migraine and signal that it is coming. These symptoms include food cravings, neck stiffness, frequent yawning, increased thirst and urination, and mood changes that range from depression to euphoria.
2. The aura stage may occur before or during the actual headache and usually lasts less than an hour. Auras usually involve visual disturbances such as flashes of light, bright spots, or a temporary blurring or loss of vision. Other signs may

include weakness or numbness in the face, hearing strange sounds, difficulty speaking, tingling sensations, muscle weakness, or paralysis to one area or one side of the body. Occasionally, the aura stage may be so severe that it can be misdiagnosed as a stroke.

3. The headache attack stage can last from a few hours to three days. During the attack, the person can experience severe throbbing head pain; nausea and vomiting; blurred vision; sensitivity to light, sound, smell and/or touch; or light-headedness and fainting. It is noteworthy that many people report a complete cessation of migraine headaches after vomiting at this stage.
4. The post-drome phase occurs after the headache attack subsides. For about a day, people experience fatigue/exhaustion, sensitivity to light and sound, confusion, dizziness, and moodiness.

Common triggers that bring on migraines include smelling certain odors like strong chemicals, continued exposure to bright or fluorescent light, severe dehydration, over-consumption of processed foods, and the biggest of them all—stress. There are no blood tests, scans, or other specific ways to determine whether a person is suffering from migraines.

Traditional treatment usually consists of over-the-counter or prescription medications aimed at mitigating the intensity of the headaches and other related symptoms. Lifestyle changes, such as eating a healthier diet, exercise, and stress-reducing activities such as yoga and meditation, appear to play a role in preventing or lessening the severity of migraines. Applied Kinesiology practitioners have discovered that restoring proper motion to the bones of the skull can successfully relieve migraine pain in most people.

* * *

LEAH, 22, was a recent college graduate who just started work in the accounting department of a movie studio. It was a stressful position, but she really enjoyed the work. However, she was concerned about her ability to keep the job, due to the fact that she suffered from frequent migraine attacks. She had experienced debilitating migraines three to four times a month since she was eighteen years old. She required four medications just to function, prescribed by doctors who specialized in migraine treatment. Due to her condition, she was forced to live at home and had attended a local college instead of going away as she had wanted.

While recovering from one of her frequent attacks at home, a friend of her mother's mentioned that she got relief from her tension headaches from treatments by an Applied Kinesiologist. Neither Leah nor her mother, had ever heard of this kind of doctor. Her friend explained that AK specializes in *helping the body heal itself* through non-invasive, drug-free techniques. Her mother took the doctor's information. Leah agreed to give it a try.

Leah appeared very timid when she entered the doctor's office. She spoke quietly and seemed nervous. During the consultation, she stated she had suffered from migraines several times a month for years. The migraines usually lasted between one and three days, and her headaches ranged from a subjective pain rating of 8–10 (with 10 being the most severe and debilitating). Usually, the attack ended once she vomited.

Leah told the Applied Kinesiologist that over the years she had been treated by a general practitioner, neurologist, endocrinologist, psychologist, and an acupuncturist. The only physical finding was of a .9 cm mixed cystic soft tissue nodule on the left lobe of her thyroid noted on a sonogram. Since the thyroid was of normal size with hormone output levels within normal limits, the endocrinologist concluded that it did not cause or affect her migraines.

She was currently taking numerous medications that helped with the intensity of the headaches but also made her nauseous most of the time. These included divalprolex (seizure medication), cyproheptadine (anti-histamine also used for anxiety), ketorolac (nonsteroidal anti-inflammatory for pain) and promethazine (to control nausea and vomiting). Initially, she took trileptol (an antiepileptic drug) but developed a tolerance to it. Then she had taken Imitrax (a migraine specific medication), which made the headaches more severe. Leah stated that she went to a gluten-free diet six months earlier with no results. She was also starting to lose some hair. Leah shared that many smells, sounds, and lights seemed to trigger her problem. At the onset of an attack, she often felt dizziness, difficulty in chewing, and generalized face pain.

Postural and Gait Analysis were unremarkable, with the exception that Leah walked very deliberately, more like a 92-year-old woman than one 22 years of age. She almost seemed unsure of her balance. She wore glasses, and her vision was 20/200.

The doctor performed several standard neurological exams on Leah to assess the functionality of her cranial nerves. These tests included smelling a bar of soap (Cranial Nerve I); reading the Snellen Eye Chart (Cranial Nerve II); various eye movements (Cranial Nerves III, IV, VI); clenching her jaw (Cranial Nerve V); smiling (Cranial Nerve VII); hearing (Cranial Nerve VIII); and opening her mouth, sticking out her tongue, and saying "AHHH." (Cranial Nerves IX, X, XII).

After having Leah perform each of the above functions, the Applied Kinesiologist would test several muscles throughout the body immediately afterward (this was not necessary for Cranial Nerve XI, since the evaluation of this cranial nerve *is* a muscle test). In each case, the muscles connected to Leah's walking and general movement were inhibited, which explained her slow walking. The Applied Kinesiologist suspected a generalized dysfunction of the rhythmic motion of the cranium.

The doctor diagnosed that the root cause of Leah's chronic migraines was cranial hypomobility, leading to an inhibition of the vagus nerve and resulting in increased intracranial pressure. The doctor showed Leah a latex model of a skull taken from the inside of a real human skull. He illustrated how restricted cranial bones could impact the vagus nerve, which modulates pressure in and around the head as well as the other cranial nerves that control senses of smell, taste, and sight. As a result, this unregulated pressure can often build up in the skull and cause serious headaches—including migraines.

The doctor postulated that the increased emotional and postural stress (first school and now her occupation) and the anticipation of suffering through yet another migraine attack caused an unconscious tightening in the muscles of her neck and jaw, which, in turn, restricted her cranial bones leading to a buildup of intracranial pressure. Leah's experience with vomiting served to reinforce this theory. The Applied Kinesiologist explained that the vagus nerve in the head is affected by emesis (vomiting). Vomiting stimulates the mechanoreceptors in the stomach and throat (pharynx) which activates the vagus nerve and could *temporarily* stimulate the nerve to perform its other function—lowering intracranial pressure. The result was an immediate relief of her migraine. Therefore, the headache relief after vomiting represented a *clue*, not a *cure*.

Leah had never received such a thorough explanation of why she was suffering from migraines. The doctor said that once the balance of pressure was restored, her condition would eventually disappear. She agreed to start the treatment immediately.

The treatment began with gentle manipulation of the various cranial bones with special attention paid to the two bones on the roof of the mouth and the mastoid bone behind her ears. The doctor then proceeded to use gentle percussion therapy over various points where several cranial bones meet, most notably just under the *glabella* between the eyes, over the *asterion* near the back of the head, and over the *pterion*. The pterion is the thinnest part of the skull on the side of the head near the temple area. It is the junction where four cranial bones join together, and Applied Kinesiologists have found that releasing tension in this area relieves pressure behind the eyes and along the sides of the head. All of these techniques are aimed at relieving intracranial pressure throughout the skull by restoring cranial bone mobility; the lack of which had led to the dysfunction of the vagus nerve.

Leah was given meditation exercises wherein she would breathe in with her tongue touching the roof of the mouth just behind the incisors to reset her cranial respiratory mechanism each day. She took the herb feverfew, which functional muscle testing revealed would be beneficial, and was advised to keep the supplement melatonin handy, in case of an attack.

After one month of biweekly treatments, Leah's attacks became less frequent, less debilitating, and shorter in duration. Gait Analysis now revealed a steadier stride and faster cadence to her walk. She consulted with her physicians about weaning her off the powerful medications that she had been taking. At first, they were reluctant but seeing how her condition was so greatly improved, they agreed. During subsequent visits to her AK professional, she reported that she had more energy and appetite. After 6 months, she was completely drug-free, and her chronic migraines had disappeared. She continues her treatments once every three months and is enjoying her life—free from the constant threat of headache pain.

TENSION-TYPE HEADACHES (TTH)

Tension-type headaches, often called stress headaches, represent the most common primary headache disorder occurring in 75% of the general adult population of the United States.[49] This condition ranges from a simple headache, due to some stressful event, to a series of painful headaches occurring close to one another. The actual physiological cause of TTH is not known, although there are factors that often contribute to it. It is usually associated with stress-related musculoskeletal problems in the neck, cranium, or jaw (TMJ), the effects of chronic poor posture, sleep deprivation, poor diet, dehydration, smoking, emotional stress, eye troubles, alcohol consumption, caffeine, and excessive time in front of a computer screen.

TTH pain is described as dull pressure around the forehead, scalp, or on the sides of the head. It is said that it feels like a belt is tightening around the skull. These headaches can last from thirty minutes to a week. Some people experience the sensation of pressure on the face, head, or neck as well as increased sensitivity to light and sound. There are no diagnostic tests to confirm TTH. Routine treatments seek only to help cope with the pain, not cure the underlying factors that may be the cause of the headaches themselves.

Over-the-counter medications such as acetaminophen, ibuprofen, or naproxen; hot pack on the head or neck; hot showers; meditation; or other relaxation techniques can ease the symptoms. However, AK has discovered that the principal cause of TTH is muscular in origin and, in most instances, can cure them and prevent the recurrence of these headaches.

* * *

DIVYA, 48, managed her husband's online nutritional company, as well as the busy lives of her two teenage sons. As her oldest son entered his junior year in high school, the college preparation activities, in addition to her other activities, started to overwhelm her. She began to get serious tension headaches daily, which often affected her work schedule.

Divya tried various nutritional supplements that had helped many of their customers, including magnesium and B vitamins. Unfortunately, they did not help in her case. Desperate for relief, she tried over-the-counter medications which helped at first, but her headaches continued. She noticed that only hot packs on the back of her neck or hot showers helped with the pain. But the headaches continued. She also experienced the attendant symptoms of nausea, dizziness, and ringing in the ears (tinnitus).

She visited her family doctor who, after an examination, diagnosed Divya with tension headaches. He suggested that she take over-the-counter medications. She informed her doctor that she had already tried them all with minimal effect and the headaches continued. Also, Divya shared that she was also experiencing nausea, dizziness, and ringing in the ears (tinnitus). Concerned about these additional symptoms, which were not generally related to TTH, her doctor ordered an MRI to rule out pathology in the brain. The family and her doctor breathed a sigh of relief when the tests came back negative.

In the follow-up consultation after the MRI, Divya related that taking the over-the-counter medications seemed to make her headaches worse rather than relieving the pain. The doctor stated that this is called a *rebound headache,* or a medication-overuse headache. Ironically, if people stop taking the medications, these rebound headaches will often subside. He told her to stop the medications, and when she did, much of her headache pain along with nausea and dizziness abated. However, she still suffered from the original headaches, and the ringing in the ears persisted.

The doctor said that he could prescribe some more powerful drugs to help with the pain, but they might make her drowsy and would not help her other symptoms. Both agreed that this did not seem to be the best solution. Because she said that so much of her tension seemed to be in her neck, her doctor suggested that Divya try chiropractic care. It often helped with tension-related conditions. He referred her to a doctor who also specialized in AK, which works the muscles safely and scientifically to help relieve tension. They took the doctor's advice and made an appointment.

The Applied Kinesiologist consulted with Divya about her stress-filled life, her hours in front of the computer, lack of exercise, and the details of her headache condition and other symptoms. He reviewed the records and MRI report and agreed with the general diagnosis of tension headaches.

Gait and Postural Analysis revealed that Divya held her shoulders high as if she was carrying weights in both hands, indicating tightness of the upper trapezius muscles that connect from the shoulder to the back of the head. Her range of cervical (neck) motion was limited, and when she looked down, she winced in pain.

The examination began with the doctor testing her upper trapezius muscles; they appeared to function normally. He then had her "stretch" these muscles, then tested them to find that they displayed a considerable dysfunction. In AK, when stretching causes a physiological weakness to a muscle, this indicates a restriction of the fascial covering of the tested muscle or a trigger point. Upper trapezius muscles are prone to this condition that can often cause severe headaches as well as ringing in the ears. Poor posture, improper ergonomics during sustained periods spent sitting at a computer, dehydration, and chronic muscle tensing due to emotional stress contribute to this dysfunction as well.

Divya was subject to most of these factors. In particular, all the additional hours that she spent on the computer managing the business, helping her son in preparation for college entrance exams and applications to various colleges, along with the emotional stress of it all, contributed to her muscular dysfunction.

The doctor continued by using Therapy Localization and range of motion studies to discover subluxations of her occiput and first cervical vertebra. These spinal misalignments can further exacerbate TTH because the lack of vertebral motion not only perpetuates the muscle spasm of the upper trapezius, which referred (sent pain) to the back of the neck and head but also decreases the activity of the joint mechanoreceptors. This leads to improper nerve impulses to the brain and stagnation of blood in the area, perpetuating the pain cycle. Lastly, the doctor tested Divya's neck muscles immediately after having her stare at her hand for ten seconds. These muscles became physiologically inhibited, indicating that Divya was suffering from weakness of her eye muscles.

After the examination concluded, he shared with Divya that her headaches originated from the extreme tension in her shoulder muscles and neck. This was the reason that the only thing that provided a short respite from her pain was heat. It facilitated the blood flow to the muscles to temporarily relax them, but they remained dysfunctional due to the tightened fascial covering. He said her treatment would begin with a deep tissue release to the fascia of the upper trapezius muscles, performed by a licensed massage therapist (LMT) attached to his practice.

Then the AK doctor applied precise spinal adjustments to the misaligned occipital and cervical bones to restore normal motion to the suboccipital area of the neck and head. Divya felt an immediate release of pressure in the back of her head and neck as well as a noticeable relaxation of her shoulders.

Afterward, the doctor showed Divya some specific exercises that she could do at home to help with her condition. He taught her some safe neck stretches to keep tension from accumulating in the back of her neck. An especially important stretch involved pushing her elbows down into the arms of the chair to counteract the common habit of raising the shoulders when working at the computer. Also, he showed her an isokinetic exercise to strengthen the muscles in the front of her neck as well. He explained that sometimes the best way to relax a chronically tight muscle is to contract and strengthen the muscle opposite in function to it. This is known as *reciprocal inhibition* and is very useful in maintaining structural corrections and keeping tension out of a compromised muscle.

Also, Divya received instructions about eye exercises to strengthen the various muscles that move the eyes, as well as those responsible for focusing on objects off in the distance and up close. He instructed her to do these three times a week along with her other strengthening exercises. The doctor also suggested she start taking extracts of the fruit bilberry as well as the herbal supplement eyebright daily, both highly effective for eye health and decreasing eye strain.

Divya required three treatments weekly for the first two weeks and then once a week for the next six weeks. By the second visit, her headaches had diminished in frequency and strength by 50%. By the end of the treatment period, they had completely disappeared along with all the other symptoms. She diligently does her neck flexor and eye exercises, along with the neck stretches, and has made strides in reducing her time in front of the computer, as well as managing her stress concerning her son's college applications.

Cluster Headaches

Cluster Headaches are among the most serious of the primary headache disorders. They can be more severe in nature than migraines. As the name suggests, they involve a grouping of headache attacks usually occurring close to each and lasting several weeks. This condition is characterized by brief but extremely painful headaches that usually focus in or around one eye and come on suddenly and continue in waves. At their worst, they can last several hours at a time. Continual and extreme stress, overconsumption of alcohol, and smoking are among the known triggers.

Cluster headaches have been called the "suicide headache" because it is the most severe of the headache conditions, and people have been known to kill themselves during an attack or in anticipation of one. They are also known as *histamine headaches* because researchers have found high levels of histamine in the person's blood and urine after a cluster attack. Histamines are natural chemicals that help dilate blood vessels to facilitate blood flow. An imbalance of histamines can increase the fluid pressure in the head and give the sufferer the impression that their heads are about to explode.

The actual cause of cluster headaches is not well understood by traditional medicine. The usual medical treatments for this condition include an injection of sumatriptan (a migraine drug) and oxygen therapy through a facemask for twenty minutes. The inhalation of pure oxygen reduces cluster headache symptoms by restricting the blood flow to the brain and decreasing the pressure inside the skull along with the pain it causes. Additional treatments include other migraine or epileptic drugs, lithium, prednisone and, occasionally, the prescription drug verapamil, which is generally used to reduce hypertension. Understanding the role of the vagus nerve in lowering intracranial pressure, the FDA has recently approved a hand-held, noninvasive vagus nerve stimulator for adjunctive use in the prevention of cluster headaches in adults; this is in addition to its previous approval of this device for migraines.[50]

Functional medical experts have found that the best way to restore normal impulses to the vagus nerve, as well as the other nerves contained within the skull, is by freeing the skull of cranial bone restrictions. It is the experience of Applied Kinesiologists that cluster headaches appear to be linked to a neurovascular condition involving a dysfunction of the main sensory nerve of the face—the trigeminal cranial nerve. When this nerve is impacted, the trigeminal-autonomic reflex pathway in the brainstem can lead to the intense headaches and eye pain associated with this serious condition.

The trigeminal nerve (Cranial Nerve V) goes through an opening in the skull (pterygopalatine fossa) made between three bones: maxilla, palatine (comprises the roof of your mouth, hence the word *palate*), and the sphenoid to enter the eye. Applied Kinesiologists have learned through clinical trials that the sphenoid bone can tilt due to tension from the jaw muscles and/or a chronic postural distortion of the head. This can affect the trigeminal nerve along with various eye nerves and the optic artery that pierce through this bone—causing pain and eye problems.

AK seeks to restore normal cranial function and relieve the problem in the neuro-muscular-skeletal complex of the head to treat and cure the underlying cause of cluster headaches.

* * *

OLEG, 35, was the CEO of a successful branding company. He worked long hours, traveled extensively, and enjoyed more than a few glasses of wine daily. As pressures of his business life increased, he started to experience severe headaches. At first, he assumed that they were stress related, and he took some over-the-counter medications to relieve the pain. However, the headaches continued to increase in frequency and intensity until the pain became intense; he lost days from work until the headaches subsided. He went to a series of doctors seeking relief. MRI, CT scan, and lumbar puncture studies were performed to rule out pathologies such as brain tumor, meningitis, or underlying sinus infection (usually more acute and accompanied by fever). All tests came back normal.

Diagnosed with cluster headaches, they gave him oxygen therapy, a variety of powerful pharmaceuticals designed for migraines, intranasal anesthetics, and a nerve block anesthetic injected into the back of the head—none of these were successful. One specialist suggested that he may need a surgical procedure known as occipital nerve stimulation, which involves implanting an electrode to stimulate the brain and the occipital nerve. Oleg was miserable. Nothing seemed to be able to relieve his condition, and he definitely did not want to undergo brain surgery.

During a visit to his brother, Oleg had a blindingly severe attack. He had to lie down in a darkened room for 12 hours until it passed. His brother was worried about him. When he found out that Oleg had been suffering these headaches for a sustained period and that all his efforts to find relief had failed, he suggested that he seek out another approach. He suggested that Oleg consider making an appointment with a doctor who had helped him deal with some serious back pain due to stress. He practiced AK, a totally unique discipline that focused on helping the body heal itself without drugs or surgery. Since he had tried nearly everything else, he agreed to give AK a try.

After Oleg finished filling out the patient profile, he joined the doctor in the consultation room. The doctor read the history and could see that besides the cluster headaches, he suffered from some vision complaints, consumed too much alcohol, and was slightly overweight. He listened while Oleg detailed his experiences with the headaches. While he talked, the doctor noticed a disparity in the openings of Oleg's eyes; his right eye looked half the size of his left. This is a common trait in patients with severe headaches.

Postural Analysis displayed that Oleg stood with his head tilted slightly to the left, and his right shoulder dropped down. Gait Analysis revealed the same imbalance of his head and shoulder.

Upon further questioning, the doctor uncovered that Oleg habitually carried his laptop computer in a bag on his right shoulder. He happened to have brought the bag to the office. The doctor walked over and picked up the bag to feel its weight. It was well beyond the weight that is healthy to carry on the same shoulder habitually.

The examination began with FMT, which displayed physiological inhibition of his right upper trapezius. The frequent pressure on the upper trapezius muscle from Oleg's bag caused the Golgi tendon organs (GTOs), the mechanoreceptors located in a muscle that measure tension, to physiologically inhibit the muscle to compensate for the strain. This dysfunction can produce a domino effect on the bones of the skull, especially the sphenoid bone that make up the floor and sides of the eye sockets, and can lead to restriction and increased pressure on pain-sensitive structures in the head.

The examination continued with Oleg lying face up on the table. The doctor had him close his eyes and gently ran the narrow end of a reflex hammer over his face. After performing this procedure, the Applied Kinesiologist, tested a neck flexor muscle (sternocleidomastoid) and a shoulder muscle (pectoralis major clavicular) immediately afterward. Both displayed functional weaknesses.

The doctor concluded that Oleg was suffering from abnormal pressure on the trigeminal cranial nerve, due to a misalignment of several skull bones, which were caused, in part, by the dysfunction of the Golgi tendon organs of the right upper trapezius muscle.

This increased skull pressure affected the brain, as well as the other cranial nerves emanating from the brain and brain stem, causing his cluster headaches.

The doctor said the treatment would involve precise adjustments to restore normal positioning of the misaligned bones, muscle manipulation therapy to the related muscles, and nutritional support to alleviate the resultant inflammation.

Before starting the mechanical corrections to the patient's cranial bones, the doctor had Oleg taste a supplement containing perilla and quercetin, natural sources of "antihistamines." He then performed the same sensation tests on Oleg's face simultaneously with the neural stimulation of tasting these nutrients. This time, the previously tested muscles remained physiologically strong. This indicated that there was an imbalance of the histamine levels, which contributed to his pain and pressure and are common in cluster headaches.

The AK specialist began by exerting gentle pressure on the junction of the maxilla/zygomatic bones in the front of his patient's face and then the maxilla/palatine bones underneath his eyes. During the second procedure, Oleg mentioned that he could feel the pain intensify behind his eye. The doctor instructed him to close his eyes and breathe deeply. Within thirty seconds of maintaining the manipulation, Oleg said that he could feel the pain and pressure behind his eye fade away.

The doctor then pushed up on the sphenoid bone which was tender. This indicated abnormal tension due to misalignment and hypertonicity (spasm) of the jaw muscles that connect there. The doctor gently manipulated these tight muscles and then the tilted sphenoid bone to restore normalcy to the eye sockets and the pterygopalatine fossa, the space through which the trigeminal nerve passes. Afterward, the doctor facilitated neural control to the upper trapezius with precise muscle manipulation to the Golgi tendon receptors—located above the shoulder blade and under the occipital bone at the back of the head. This would help ensure that Oleg's head and cranial bones remain level and free of compression.

After the gentle correction to Oleg's cranial structure, the doctor suggested that he come in twice a week for a month to ensure the sustained correction of his cranial bones, in order to maintain proper functioning of his cranial nerves, and to relax and restore balance to the trapezius muscles as well as his jaw and eye muscles. Oleg was instructed to change from a shoulder bag to a backpack to distribute weight more evenly between his shoulders and invest in a lighter laptop. The doctor also suggested that Oleg address his stress levels with meditation and classical music, change his diet, lose weight, cut back on the wine, and take the natural antihistamine supplement that he had tasted during the treatment. After two months of treatments and his diligent attention to the recommended lifestyle changes, he has never had another attack.

* * *

Traditional medicine treats headache disorders with drugs and therapies that help the patient cope with the pain until the headaches subside on their own. It does not acknowledge the underlying functional origins of this disorder and tends to deal with the symptoms only.

Fortunately, integrative medicine specialists using AK FMT and other diagnostic tools have found that the primary cause of most headaches are usually located within the mechanics of the interlocking and interdependent cranial bones as well as the supporting cervical spine and related nerves and muscles, which can lead to increased pressure within your skull (idiopathic intracranial hypertension). This increase in pressure can create various types of headaches, depending upon the part of the brain, brainstem or cranial nerves most affected.

Once pathology has been ruled out, AK therapy can begin the healing process of freeing up any biomechanical restrictions within the skull and cervical spine and help regulate the nerve impulses, normalize blood flow, and induce the brain lymphatics to drain from the cranium. For this reason, doctors trained in AK generally have good success in relieving most forms of headaches.

15

PSYCHO-PHYSIOLOGICAL CONDITIONS

Psychological conditions such as attention deficit hyperactivity disorder (ADHD), depression, anxiety, seasonal affective disorder (SAD), phobias, dyslexia, broken-heart syndrome, performance anxiety, post-traumatic stress disorder (PTSD), self-sabotage or fear of success syndrome, and a host of others can have a tremendous impact on your health. These conditions can affect every aspect of a person's life and lead to serious physical problems including heart conditions, ulcers, hypertension, and drug abuse. Traditional medicine usually approaches these conditions using some combination of psychotherapeutic and/or prescribed medications with varying degrees of success.

Conspicuously lacking in the treatment of emotional conditions is *psycho-physiological* therapy. Applied Kinesiology emphasizes the body-mind or soma-psychic connection in its approach to treating these disorders by addressing specific physical problems that may be manifesting as emotional symptoms. In many cases, the source of the condition can be traced to a functional imbalance in the body, often involving some kind of impacted neural feedback. The condition can affect a variety of systems, including the brain and hormonal systems. Once the source of the physiological problem is found and treated, the soma-psychic balance of the body can be restored, and the patient can find relief from his or her emotional difficulties. Applied Kinesiology has several unique procedures to address the *physiological* aspect of psycho-physiological conditions specifically. Three such modalities are Neurological Disorganization Syndrome correction, Anxiety Release Procedure, and Emotional Recall Technique.

Applied Kinesiologists have isolated a physical condition that can be at the root of many disorders perceived to be purely emotional in nature: *Neurological Disorganization Syndrome* (NDS). This condition is difficult for traditional medicine to diagnose and is often overlooked, much in the same way that *pre-menstrual syndrome* and *post-partum depression* used to be. While its symptoms and their effects on health are concrete and definable, it is not acknowledged as a medical condition because it defies traditional categorization.

Neurological Disorganization Syndrome is linked to many conditions such as anxiety attacks, attention deficit disorder (ADD), learning disabilities, behavioral disorders, dyslexia, hyperactivity, attention deficit hyperactivity disorder (ADHD), and PTSD. Correcting NDS could help lessen their overall psychological effects on the individual. Neurological Disorganization Syndrome is also commonly found to be an underlying contributing factor to short-term memory loss and disorientation in seniors. To have a better understanding of NDS and how to correct it, we need to have a clear understanding of how the nervous system works.

Your nervous system has three general functions: a *sensory function* to receive information, an *interpretive function* to process this information, and a *motor function* to transmit the processed information. Essentially, sensory (afferent) nerves gather information from the internal and external environment and deliver this information to your central nervous system (CNS). This received information is processed, interpreted, and transmitted through motor (efferent) nerves from the CNS to the approximately 650 muscles and 78 glands and organs in your body. Neurological disorganization syndrome is what occurs when there is a physiological problem interrupting the proper functioning of this neural network.

The central nervous system (brain and spinal cord) is the *integration and command center* of the body. The unconscious processing capabilities of your brain are estimated to be 11 million pieces of information per second; whereas, your conscious processing capabilities are estimated to be about 50 pieces of information per second.[51] This large disparity in capacity means that, while processing the constant influx of these signals, a single physical or emotional trauma or the cumulative effects of chronic stress can cause the conscious system to "overload." As a result, the CNS will try to protect itself by "powering down" some of its processing capabilities. This is similar to the way the Golgi tendon organ mechanoreceptors in a particular muscle will inhibit the function of that muscle to prevent it from tearing or suffering a serious pathological problem. Our bodies appear to have built-in, fail-safe mechanisms to delay or prevent a wide variety of physical dysfunctions. Neurological disorganization syndrome represents a *psychological-physiological* disruption of that fail-safe mechanism brought on by stress overload.

NDS manifests in a variety of subtle but significant ways such as jumbling words, moodiness, difficulty with directions, short-term memory lapses, performance failures on tests or in routine activities, semi-grogginess, disorientation, transposing of numbers, and fatigue. More serious symptoms involve depression, anxiety, sudden bursts of anger, and violent and self-destructive behavior including suicidal tendencies. Once successfully diagnosed and treated, these complaints will become less intrusive or disappear completely.

Occasionally, some patients will experience lingering physical injuries like an ankle sprain that is inexplicably not healing as it should due to NDS. In other cases, this neural *processing* disturbance manifests as a physiological dysfunction of a muscle on the side opposite to where the doctor would expect it (motor manifestation), or the patient senses pain in a seemingly healthy area (sensory manifestation)—both due to NDS.

Of the varied conditions that your AK doctor is able to help you with, none may be more powerful and life-affirming than correcting NDS. This is because NDS can affect nearly every system in the body. For example, when the *sensory* part of your nervous system is affected, you might experience symptoms such as pain or numbness. When the *motor* part of your nervous system is affected, you may experience muscular weakness or spasms as well as endocrine, breathing or digestive problems. When the *processing* aspect of your nervous system is afflicted, it can create a baffling array of vague or sometimes painful "symptoms" that are difficult to diagnose because there is no obvious cause.

Neurological disorganization syndrome can be corrected by reducing the overall level of stress your nervous system is contending with, most often due to dysfunction of the cranial bones, TMJ, and other improperly aligned structures whose improper movement creates a barrage of mechanoreceptor (pressure) or nociceptor (pain) signals that disrupt your neural perceptual and processing abilities.

An illustration of sensory manifestation of this *processing* dysfunction is witnessed in the case of a woman who suffered a left-sided rib injury after falling off a horse. The emergency room took X-rays, ruled out a fracture and diagnosed her with bruised left ribs. She visited her Applied Kinesiologist, who did gentle muscle manipulation and ultrasound therapy over the area to speed healing. A few days later, she returned to say that she had no pain over her left ribcage but was experiencing the pain on the right side.

The doctor could find no explanation for this. Suspecting NDS, the doctor examined her to find that she had become *neurologically disorganized*, in all likelihood, due to the overstimulation of her nervous system from the intense pain after her fall. When the doctor performed gentle cranial manipulation therapy to the patient's skull, the pain disappeared instantaneously on the right side and reverted back to her left. The patient was amazed by how her pain could simply *switch* sides. The doctor explained that pain signals are only *carried* by nerves (nociceptors), but it is the brain that *interprets* these signals. In this patient's case, her neural processing system had been disrupted by the trauma of her fall, and the intense pain that she felt afterward caused her brain to interpret the pain signals as coming from the right side instead of the left. Once the *switching* (NDS) was corrected, the doctor continued with therapy to increase circulation to help heal the bruised left rib.

Along with correcting NDS, your Applied Kinesiologist has additional technical tools such as The Anxiety Release Procedure which is effective in treating some of the *physical* causes related to depression, phobias, performance anxiety, and self-sabotaging behaviors. It is a technique that integrates visualization with acupuncture procedures to help dampen excessive nervousness and the overreaction to certain situations, such as a fear of flying or public speaking, caused by a blockage in the energy meridians of the body. This technique, developed by a psychologist who specialized in AK, has been so successful in its outcomes that it is sometimes affectionately known as "The 5-Minute Phobia Cure."

The Emotional Recall Technique is a time-proven procedure that lessens the physiological reactions to past trauma through precise stimulation of skin mechanoreceptors on your forehead. These skin mechanoreceptors are under the control of the fifth cranial nerve, which is the largest of the cranial nerves and also controls the TMJ muscles. This includes the powerful masseter muscle—the muscle most often involved in cases of stress-induced jaw clenching. Applied Kinesiologists have found that stimulating these mechanoreceptors over the frontal bone while the patient is concentrating on the memory of a stressful situation appears to have a calming *physiological* effect on *psychological* stress. People suffering from PTSD are an example of individuals who have been helped by this, and other AK procedures, that restore the psycho-physiological balance.

While potent and powerfully effective, these three techniques are not designed to replace psychotherapy but rather augment it by addressing the physiological factors that may be contributing to or exacerbating emotional problems. Once these factors are addressed and cured, psychotherapy can be more effective.

Attention Deficit Hyperactivity Disorder (ADHD)

Attention Deficit Hyperactivity Disorder (ADHD) is a mental/behavioral disorder characterized by an inability to maintain attention accompanied by impulsive behavior and hyperactivity. In people with ADHD, chemicals in the brain called neurotransmitters are not as active in parts of the brain that control the ability to focus attention. Researchers do not know what exactly causes this neurological imbalance. There is no single test to diagnose ADHD. However, a series of computer-based tasks that measure attention and problem-solving skills can reveal the principal traits of this condition in conjunction with a patient's behavioral history. The three main types of ADHD are the primarily inattentive type, primarily hyperactive-impulsive type, and combined type.

ADHD is commonly diagnosed in children with behaviors including trouble sitting still, completing tasks, following directions, and socially disruptive behavior. Nearly one in six boys in the U.S under the age of 10 and an estimated 11% of all children have been diagnosed with ADHD.[52] Some experts believe that this rate of diagnosis is too high, yet it seems to be growing. It is estimated that 30-70% of children with ADHD continue to have symptoms as adults even after treatment.[53]

Signs of ADHD in adults include habitually running late, easily distracted and an inability to stay focused on the task at hand, risky driving, problems with self-control, impulsive actions, difficulty controlling anger, blurting out inappropriate or rude comments, constant need to be stimulated, and inability to follow through with routine tasks. Adults with ADHD tend to struggle with anxiety, depression, and obsessive-compulsive disorder (OCD) and are more likely to engage in activities that distract them from their symptoms, such as overuse of alcohol, drugs, and tobacco.

Traditional medical treatments for ADHD in both children and adults usually involve a combination of behavioral therapy and some form of medication. Often it can be a slippery slope with adjustments in the type and dosage of drugs that can leave the patient in a constant state of flux, often making their condition worse.

* * *

SUNNY, 8, was a bright and engaging girl who had been having trouble in school. She had difficulty with comprehension, as well as with completing assignments in class. It was difficult for her to sit still and remain quiet. Her family was not native English speakers, so English was not her first language. Teachers initially thought her difficulties were in part due to the possibility that she simply did not fully understand what her teachers were asking of her. However, as she got older, it became evident something else was going on. Her grades were too low for a child of her obvious intelligence and abilities. Her parents noticed her restlessness at home but thought that she was just a particularly energetic child. They encouraged her to play sports, such as soccer, to burn up her excess energy.

At a parent-teacher meeting, the homeroom teacher stated in her evaluation that, "Sunny was social, creative, kind and 'always full of smiles' but had issues with her focus, attention, impulsivity, and high activity level." Sunny's other teachers related in writing that she "required, constant re-direction and occasional reprimanding." Her parents had heard these kinds of comments over the years about their daughter's behavior but thought that they were just part of Sunny's personality; yet, they couldn't understand why her grades were so low.

However, it seemed that her classroom behavior was getting more and more disruptive, so her teachers suggested that Sunny see the school psychologist. After reviewing her record and observing her, she offered an initial diagnosis of ADHD. She suggested that her parents discuss the possibility of therapy and medications to help their daughter's condition and improve her performance in school by seeing a psychiatrist specializing in ADHD. If Sunny's behavior did not improve, she might have to be placed in a special class. Realizing the gravity of Sunny's condition, they agreed to have her see a specialist.

The specialist conducted a full psychological evaluation which revealed mental processing difficulties, attention deficit, hyperactivity, headaches, visual disturbances, and hearing difficulties. The doctor concluded that Sunny suffered from combined-type ADHD complicated by Sunny's other physical issues. He suggested that Sunny be tested for visual and hearing impairment and begin behavioral therapy with sixty-two items to be addressed at home and in the classroom. If her behavior did not improve, he recommended medication. Sunny and her parents attempted to follow these measures but found them too overwhelming.

Also, an ophthalmologist examined Sunny's complaints of eye strain (asthenopia), "seeing double," headaches, and an *eyebrow-ache* over the left eye while reading or performing prolonged tasks. The examination revealed that she experienced an *intermittent exotropia* (eye misalignment), a condition in which your eyes do not work together when looking at nearby objects. Visual acuity on a Snellen eye chart displayed a visual acuity of 20/25 in each eye. The doctor did not feel glasses were needed and prescribed eye muscle/orthoptic exercises. While Sunny liked the exercises and was diligent in doing them, they did not improve her vision.

Lastly, an otolaryngologist performed a comprehensive hearing exam, including audiometry and tympanometry tests, to address Sunny's complaint that sometimes she could not hear instructions in class. These tests revealed Sunny to have mild hearing loss in the left ear, which the doctor felt could contribute to her inability to comprehend instructions and her resultant frustration.

Overwhelmed by the findings of the three specialists, Sunny's parents didn't know what to do. They wanted Sunny to succeed but were reluctant to put her on what could be a lifetime of drug therapy. They had a friend whose son had suffered from ADHD as a boy but seemed to be fine now. He attended college and was doing well. Sunny's father discussed this situation with their old friend. He commiserated with him, having gone through many of the same experiences with doctors that Sunny's family had. On the advice of a friend, he had taken their son to a doctor that specialized in AK. After a series of treatments, his son's condition became increasingly manageable without any medications until he barely had any problems. Sunny's dad took the information and immediately made an appointment.

The Applied Kinesiologist reviewed the records, including the in-depth 30-page psychiatrist's Neuropsychological/Psychoeducational Evaluation as well as the eye and hearing exams. Intrigued by the pattern of Sunny's headaches, eyebrow pain, and hearing deficit—all occurring on the left side of her head—the doctor asked if there had been any head trauma. The parents recalled that a few years earlier, Sunny fell on her head doing gymnastics. Though it was nothing serious, they switched her to playing soccer—which, thus far, had been without any major incident aside from her falling down frequently.

Standard neurological tests revealed no deficit in Sunny's reactions. Postural Analysis was normal. However, Gait Analysis revealed that Sunny's arms and legs did not work in the normal way. Instead of her arms and legs moving smoothly with the right arm and left leg moving forward and in the same pattern using the opposite limbs (known as the alternative reciprocal pattern found in normal walking), they moved with the arm and leg on the *same* side moving simultaneously, creating a forced and unnatural movement pattern.

The examination proceeded with Sunny lying on the table for a few minutes while the doctor asked some questions that she could not answer due to a lack of focus. Sunny, intrigued by the mechanical examination table that moved up and down, asked a series of questions of her own in rapid succession. The doctor was happy to provide answers and then proceeded to test random neck, shoulder, and hip muscles; they all measured physiologically strong.

The doctor continued the examination by having Sunny come up off the table and walk up and down the hall for a minute. Then she resumed her face-up position on the table, and the doctor immediately tested the exact same set of muscles. This time, manual muscle testing revealed profound physiological weakness of every muscle tested. The act of walking usually supported the function of the nervous system, but in Sunny's case, it seemed to have disrupted the mechanoreceptors in key muscles which could affect her overall neural processing of information, especially visual and auditory, and lead to her other behaviors.

The brain is not rigid, and nerves are not static wires that simply conduct electrical impulses. They both have what is called *neuroplasticity*, meaning that your brain and nervous system adapt to form new connections and pathways when stimulated to do so. These new pathways allow us to perform tasks at a more refined level, as they allow actions to go from requiring conscious execution initially to developing into a subconscious automatic function.

AK treatments can improve this neuroplasticity by removing physiological impediments to the nervous system, thereby restoring proper processing of information. In many people (especially children) diagnosed with learning disabilities, dyslexia, or ADHD, this dysfunctional processing of information is often the root cause of their behavior.

After a minute of resting on the table, Sunny had regained her normal physiological muscle function, and the doctor proceeded with the exam. He had Sunny crisscross her arms and placed them over her chest (Therapy Localize) on the part of the skin that is controlled by the first thoracic spinal segment. This spinal segment is the origin of the sympathetic nervous system. He tested her muscle function. Each muscle tested became physiologically inhibited while she maintained this position. AK practitioners have found that this particular inhibition can indicate NDS.

The doctor continued to muscle test and found that Sunny had cranial restrictions of her occipital, temporal, sphenoid, and frontal bones—as well as the muscles of her jaw (TMJ) that may have initially occurred from landing on her head in gymnastics. In all likelihood, this restriction of the natural movement of her skull bones caused NDS, which resulted in the lack of coordination that subsequently led to Sunny's frequent falls while playing soccer; that, in turn, reinforced the cranial bone restrictions. Over the years, these cranial bone restrictions could have been contributing to the improper processing of information in the cerebrum, cerebellum, and brainstem, as well as being the cause of her "eyebrow pain" and headaches.

Additional functional muscle tests also revealed a dysfunction of specific brain-related skin mechanoreceptors (neurolymphatic receptors). These "brain points" are located on the front of the body near the shoulder, slightly below the coracoid process of the shoulder blade and posterior to the transverse process of the atlas bone (first cervical vertebra) just under the skull in the back of the neck. Congestion of these specific skin receptors has been postulated to impede the proper drainage of lymphatic waste out of the brain and can lead to many of the same symptoms attributed to ADHD. Although only recently discovered, these lymphatic vessels appear to carry waste out of the cerebrospinal fluid in the brain into the cervical lymph nodes in the neck, where they can be filtered out of the body.

After concluding all these tests, the doctor shared that Sunny's symptoms of ADHD and her visual and auditory issues apparently originated with the condition called NDS. The parents looked concerned, but the doctor said that this condition was not uncommon and could be corrected with treatment and without any medications. She could begin treatments as soon as Sunny and her parents were ready.

Sunny began her weekly treatments the following week. They included gentle cranial manipulation, fascial release technique of the skull and jaw muscles, and percussion therapy over the sympathetic chain ganglion over the thoracic spine. The doctor then proceeded to manipulate the *brain lymphatic mechanoreceptors* for 30 seconds to positively stimulate the brain and free it from any potential build-up of metabolic waste.

By the end of the first treatment, Sunny was attentive and relaxed. The Applied Kinesiologist brought Sunny up off the table and had her walk down the hall. Her alternative reciprocal walking pattern seemed improved. The doctor instructed Sunny's parents to rub, with firm rotary pressure, the receptors located just below the patient's collar bone for thirty seconds every day.

After the third treatment, Sunny again performed the crisscross pattern with her arms, and this time the muscles were not inhibited or dysfunctional.

By the fifth visit, Sunny's walking pattern was completely normal. Her parents reported that she was no longer falling on the soccer field. The doctor taught Sunny and her parents a deep-breathing-walking-in-place exercise to do every morning and night with Sunny to help with her focus, balance, and coordination. The doctor also recommended that Sunny start each day with a protein-based breakfast to help brain activity.

After the sixth treatment, Sunny came home exuberant from school that week after she completed a pop quiz five minutes early. On her next visit, her mother related that this was the first time that Sunny did not come off the bus in a miserable mood and upset that she could not complete the class assignment.

After three months of treatments, Sunny's parents reported that her teachers had seen a marked difference in her performance. She was now reading at the appropriate grade level, got along with the other children, and did not display any disruptive behavior. Sunny reported her reading "blurriness" only occurred when the book was right at her nose. Vision and hearing tests were now normal, and she no longer suffered from headaches or pain over the left eyebrow.

Since her behavior and performance had improved so much, the school removed the label of ADHD from Sunny's file. The AK specialist was not surprised, since ADHD, in many cases, is more of a collection of symptoms, not primarily a psychological condition. Once the origin of the symptoms was found and treated, the condition had disappeared.

Sunny continues to be examined once a month and receives any necessary treatment. As her condition improves, she enjoys school, has more friends, and is excelling on the soccer field. Her future looks bright.

Performance Anxiety

Performance anxiety is a psycho-physical condition in which your mind creates such extreme tension in your body that you are unable to perform a task that you are quite capable of executing. Examples include faring poorly on college admissions or job interviews, freezing up when asked to speak in front of a group, playing poorly in high-pressure competitive sports, or not reaching one's potential in a profession due to the fear of failure. On a more private level, it can impede sexual intimacy in relationships as well.

Symptoms of performance anxiety include panic attacks; phobias; fainting; severe blushing; heart pounding; nausea; profuse sweating; trembling of the hands, knees, and voice; the inability to perform routine or rehearsed tasks; impotence; and other forms of extreme physical and psychological distress.

Sports psychologists have found that how you personally interpret a situation is important to your performance under so-called *pressure*. In other words, if you perceive a situation as a *challenge* your body releases adrenaline which enhances performance; however, if you interpret the same scenario as a *threat,* your body releases cortisol which impedes performance. Therefore, depending on whether you believe you are up to the task (a challenge) or if you think the task is overwhelming (a threat), plays a significant role in how you respond and ultimately perform. These performance experts conclude that it is not the task itself that determines success or failure—it is how you choose to view yourself in relation to it that does.

There is a myriad of techniques designed to help cope with performance anxiety such as meditation, visualization, and keeping the importance of the task or situation in perspective, as well as a host of medications. These all can be very effective; however, there are times that this condition may not be completely psychological. Sometimes there is a deeper physiological issue that undermines our best efforts to remain calm and focused under pressure, whether internal or external. Applied Kinesiology's *somatopsychic* approach (physical corrections to relieve psychological symptoms) to restore the balance of the mind-body connection has proved particularly successful in treating many forms of performance anxiety.

* * *

DAVID, 31, had recently risen up the ranks of the financial institution at which he worked to become a portfolio manager. He had earned his BBA degree in Finance and had become a CFA (Chartered Financial Analyst). David's life-long dream was to become a CEO of his own financial company. However, as his expertise increased, his boss wanted him to make presentations on behalf of the company to clients, analysts, and investors around the world. David was worried about his new responsibility because he suffered from a deep fear of speaking in front of a group of people. Just thinking about it would make him sweat profusely, blush, have anxiety attacks, and lose sleep.

On the eve of his first presentation, he tried to prepare himself, but the following morning he was an emotional wreck, and the presentation went badly. He tried several other times with the same results. Eventually, his boss gave the presentations to another person, and David was demoted. He knew that to progress in his career, he would have to overcome this performance anxiety about public speaking. He sought out a psychologist who specialized in performance anxiety. He took some mild anti-anxiety medications prescribed by his medical doctor. However, nothing seemed to help.

David was in excellent physical shape and enjoyed playing baseball in an adult league. It helped him manage his stress. However, sometime after his problems at work began, he developed severe pain in the elbow of his pitching arm. The orthopedist he visited said there was a Grade 1 tear of the ulnar collateral ligament. He gave him a cortisone shot and had a physical therapist perform massage, muscle stimulation, ice applications, and ultrasound therapy. After a few weeks, the pain was not any better. His doctor was surprised at his lack of progress and suggested that he have surgery to correct the problem. He couldn't afford to take time off from work, and his condition added more stress to his life. Some of the fellow players on the team went to a local doctor of chiropractic, who specialized in AK, and several of them suggested that David try it. He agreed.

After filling out the detailed patient profile, the doctor could see that David was nervous as he discussed his elbow pain and his concerns about work. The doctor asked him if he had any other related symptoms. David reported that when he was anxious, he would often experience a lump in the throat, dry mouth, nervous stomach, and occasional cold sweats.

When the doctor asked more about this array of symptoms, David stated that this was what he would feel before and during the work-related meetings or presentations. His symptoms seemed to indicate performance anxiety. The doctor told him that he may have an answer for those maladies once they fixed the elbow problem.

Postural Analysis displayed no obvious issues. Gait Analysis revealed that David did not move his shoulders and arms much when he walked; they moved so slightly that he looked like he was walking with his hands in his pockets. Range of motion studies showed David to be very stiff, especially for a young athletic man. Using a tape measure, the doctor measured how far his patient could come to touching the floor and found that David's fingers could only reach ten inches from the floor. David mentioned that, no matter how much he stretched, he was always tight. The doctor replied that "tight muscles" were often the result of underlying nervous tension.

During the examination, the Applied Kinesiologist found that what appeared to be causing the constant strain to the ulnar collateral ligament (UCL) and inflammation to the elbow tendons was a medially misaligned ulna bone, the larger of the two forearm bones. This misalignment could eventually lead to a serious tear which would require surgery. Luckily, they had caught it in time. Three weeks of treatments included chiropractic manipulation of the ulna and Origin/Insertion Technique to the forearm muscles, especially the pronator teres and the wrist flexor muscles, which have a large common tendon originating in this area. These treatments, in conjunction with the physical therapy to help relieve the inflammation of the now realigned bone, successfully relieved the joint, ligament, and tendon problem.

Then it was on to the treatment of David's performance anxiety.

The doctor had David perform some basic muscle mobility tests, such as touching his toes. He could only reach eight inches from the floor. Afterward, he had him lie face down on the treatment table and discovered a lack of motion of his spinal bones, especially between the shoulder blades. This tension can result in a low level of constant pressure on the nervous system and create the feeling of being "revved up" all of the time, a predisposition for performance anxiety. In some people, this store of "nervous energy" can be productive when channeled. In others, this feeling of being "on edge" all the time could contribute to general anxiety. David nodded, admitting he was so hyper that he would habitually bounce his leg fervently when sitting. The constant bombardment of his nervous system from the mechanoreceptors in his restricted spine and shoulder joints contributed to his constant state of nervousness, which peaked during particularly stressful situations.

Treatment to address the *physiological* aspects of David's conditions began with precise chiropractic spinal manipulation therapy to free up the restricted vertebrae, which were limiting movement of the spine between David's shoulder blades and *revving up* his nervous system. Afterward, the doctor used a deep percussion roller to go up and down both sides of the spine directly over where the sympathetic chain ganglia, also called the paravertebral ganglia, reside deep underneath the muscles on both sides of the spine. After the spinal adjustments and deep percussion therapy, the doctor had David again perform range of motion studies to assess his muscular tightness due to nervous tension. He could now touch his toes easily.

After working the spine and the paravertebral ganglia to control *generalized* nervousness, the doctor proceeded to perform an *emotional challenge* to find a *specific* trigger of David's nerves. He had David close his eyes and visualize himself speaking in a professional setting with a microphone to a group of investors. While he closed his eyes and held this picture in his mind, the doctor proceeded to test the pectoralis major clavicular, a shoulder muscle that Applied Kinesiologists have found highly correlated with *emotional stress*. The pectoralis major clavicular muscle became drastically inhibited during this visualization.

This confirmed the *psycho-physiological* origin of David's performance anxiety. Concurrently, David began to develop some other symptoms of distress while maintaining this visualization exercise. Even though he was still relaxing on the table, his face became flushed, his palms started sweating, and he began repeatedly swallowing because of tension in his throat. The doctor had David stand up and try to touch his toes again, but he could not. This confirmed the dual-edged approach necessary to address both the general physiological and specific psychological aspects of David's performance anxiety.

Functional muscle testing revealed a blockage in the acupuncture point in the *stomach meridian*, which corresponds to the emotion of *anxiety*. Treatment consisted of tapping the first and last acupuncture points of the stomach meridian forty times while David thought about a stressful situation. This rhythmic tapping technique, while a patient thinks about an emotionally stressful situation, is known in AK as the Anxiety Release Procedure.

After the AK acupuncture tapping procedure, the doctor asked David to visualize the public speaking scenario again and tested the pectoralis major clavicular muscles. This time, his muscles no longer became physiologically inhibited, his other symptoms did not appear, and he was able to touch his toes—a clear sign of decreased neural tension.

When David asked how this was possible, the doctor explained that AK functional muscle testing measures the physiological function that is often linked to psychological pressure—similar to a polygraph test that displays physiological changes due to emotional duress when someone tells a lie. The muscle testing revealed that David's muscles were physiologically influenced to function in a negative way when he pictured himself in what he perceived to be a stressful situation. Too much neural activity excessively tightened up David's entire *muscular* system, leading to additional emotional stress and physical responses such as heart palpitations, anxiety symptoms, and throat tightening. In David's case, this increased neural activity originated in a blockage of the energy meridians in his stomach, which may have affected or been affected by a lack of free motion of his spine and shoulders, thereby compounding the stress reaction. Once the blockage was taken away, the rest of his system could function normally, and his stress level would decrease.

David required six treatments in total regarding his performance anxiety and has never had another incident of uncontrollable stage fright or performance anxiety about public speaking. The doctor also supplemented David's diet with omega-3 fatty acids, since recent findings support the appearance of them having an "anti-anxiety effect." Free from the fear of these public speaking *meltdowns*, David joined Toastmasters International to develop his communication skills and became a vibrant speaker. He was approached by an institutional investor who was in his audience and was very impressed with his knowledge and vision. David is now CEO and co-founder of a financial technology company delivering blockchain solutions for global financial institutions.

Broken-Heart Syndrome

Broken heart syndrome, (Takotsubo cardiomyopathy) also known as *acute stress-induced cardiomyopathy*, is a temporary heart condition that causes sudden chest pain and mimics a heart attack. It is usually caused by an unexpected stressful situation such as the death of a loved one, major relationship breakups, financial problems, job loss, and a deep sense of betrayal. In rare cases, broken heart syndrome can be fatal.

In broken heart syndrome, there is a temporary disruption of the heart's normal pumping action usually due to the heart's reaction to a surge of adrenal stress hormones. Symptoms include chest pain and shortness of breath. It most commonly occurs in women over 50 years of age.

Broken heart syndrome is generally treated with medications such as ACE inhibitors (lowers blood pressure by working on the kidneys), beta-blockers (lowers blood pressure by working on the adrenal glands) and diuretics (lowers blood pressure by eliminating fluids). The aim of these medications is not to treat the condition but help the heart as it heals on its own. While complications can occur, most people who survive the initial shock to the heart will recuperate within two months. Applied Kinesiologists take a different approach to help your heart to heal from stress-induced conditions, including broken heart syndrome.

* * *

MEI-LIEN, 50, was the wife of a successful entrepreneur and mother of four grown children who had all recently finished college and were starting their careers. Now that her children were out of the house, she wanted to pursue her lifelong dream of starting her own aromatherapy business. Over the years, she had seen the results that aromatherapy had demonstrated in her life and wanted to help other people with it. She started the company with a partner, and it became a success. However, despite the company's growth, the revenue after the first year didn't seem to reflect the strength of the business. She contacted her accountant to analyze the books. It seemed that her partner, who was also her cousin, had been embezzling money and selling products outside of the company. Mei-Lien was devastated.

She confronted her cousin and severed all ties with her. The business faltered, and Mei-Lien worked tirelessly to keep it going. Exhausted and depressed, Mei-Lien began experiencing pains in her chest. One night, the pains become so severe that she went to the emergency room, afraid that she was having a heart attack. The emergency room doctors performed an EKG, but it came back normal. Since the pain continued, she consulted with a cardiologist, who suggested that she have a cardiac angiography to check for any serious blockages that might be causing the pain. The test came back negative for coronary artery stenosis or obstructive coronary artery disease.

Since Mei-Lien continued to have deep chest pain but no major pathology, her cardiologist diagnosed her with Takotsubo cardiomyopathy, commonly known as "broken-heart syndrome." While the exact cause of this condition is unclear, it is believed to be linked to a surge of stress hormones, such as adrenaline, and triggered by an emotionally traumatic event which could temporarily damage the heart muscle and cause pain. Most patients completely recover within one or two months with no treatment. Occasionally, doctors may prescribe medications, such as beta blockers to block the potentially damaging effects of stress hormones on the heart, and anxiety-reducing drugs. Relieved to hear that her condition was not life-threatening, she agreed to take the medications to help her heal more quickly.

However, even though Mei-Lien took the prescribed medications, she continued to suffer from pain deep in her chest, now accompanied by inexplicable fatigue. She thought that it might be linked to her depression over her cousin's betrayal, so she entered psychotherapy which helped her emotionally—but the physical symptoms lingered. The psychologist stated that she believed there was a physical issue beyond what she could help with, so she referred Mei-Lien to an acupuncturist. Mei-Lien experienced a benefit in her energy levels from acupuncture, but the effects did not last, and there was no relief of her chest pain. The acupuncturist suggested that she try a doctor she knew who specialized in AK who would be better able to find the source of her condition. She made an appointment.

Mei-Lien was sitting in the consultation room drinking hot tea when the doctor entered. He immediately noticed that she was holding the warm beverage against her chest, and it appeared to comfort her. During the consultation, Mei-Lien frequently put her fingers to her forehead (with the warm tea still pressed against her chest) while she spoke about her symptoms and the events leading up to them.

After reviewing her medical records, the doctor had Mei-Lien explain the history of her condition. She related that it had begun soon after her cousin had betrayed her and stolen from the business they had co-founded. It was a struggle for her to keep the business afloat after that, and she never got over it. Her pains started to impact her life, she fell into depression, and she suffered from fatigue. She had tried medications, acupuncture, and therapy, but still had debilitating pain. After hearing her story, the AK specialist could understand why her cardiologist had diagnosed her with Takotsubo cardiomyopathy.

He then had her engage in Postural and Gait analysis, both of which revealed her palms to be facing noticeably forward. Her shoulders were excessively rotated forward, and there was a slight curve of her thoracic spine. This condition is called *kyphosis*. Most doctors acknowledge that severe kyphosis can create breathing difficulties, as well as put pressure on the internal organs of the thoracic cavity—most notably the heart and lungs. However, it is often overlooked that even a small accentuation of the natural curve of the thoracic spine, such as in Mei-Lien's case, can create these same problems.

The examination proceeded with spinal palpation, which revealed that several of the midback spinal segments were misaligned. Functional muscle testing uncovered a physiological inhibition of the lower trapezius muscles on both sides, contributing to her slightly hunched over appearance, as well as the subscapularis muscles that rest deep under the shoulder blade. The subscapularis inhibition also explained the excessive shoulder rotation that caused her palms to face forward.

Proceeding from the back to the front, the doctor found that invoking a deep percussion upon the chest and directly over the heart created physiological facilitation of the heart-related subscapularis muscles. This positive neural response to deep percussion indicated a possible fascial restriction directly over the heart and represented the most likely cause of Mei-Lien's inexplicable deep chest pain and recurrent fatigue.

Therefore, in addition to her thoracic kyphosis, spinal subluxations, and muscular dysfunction, the doctor surmised, in Mei-Lien's case, that the physiological response to the intense psychological shock she had received caused an overall inhibition of her diaphragm muscle and altered its connection with the outer layer of the pericardium of her heart. All of this characterizes what is called *The Startle Reflex* and could create a restriction of the fascial covering over the heart (pericardium)—leading to chest pain, fatigue, and other symptoms of "broken heart syndrome."

The heart is encased in a tight covering sac called the pericardium. The pericardium has two layers: the outer coat (parietal pericardium) and the inner coat (visceral pericardium). The outer coat connects to the diaphragm and the back of the breastbone, while the inner coat has one layer that connects to the outer one and another layer that closely adheres to the heart. The space between these two layers is filled with pericardial fluid that acts as a lubricant which allows smooth movement of your heart within the chest cavity.

The doctor explained that the complex series of factors which he had discovered were placing undue pressure on her heart and other muscles in her chest. Since her medical records did not show any serious damage to the heart itself, he suggested that some chiropractic adjustive therapy, along with percussion therapy directly over the heart, could be the answer to relieving her condition. Mei-Lien nodded in agreement. The doctor proceeded to perform the precise spinal manipulation to restore normal motion to the lower thoracic spine and restore normal function to the lower trapezius muscles, as well as to the diaphragm which has connections to that specific area. He then performed a maneuver to release the upper thoracic vertebrae from their misaligned position. Mei-Lien immediately felt a dramatic relief throughout her body.

The doctor placed a percussion device over her heart to release any fascial restrictions of the pericardium. This Heart Percussion Technique has been called, "AK-CPR." After this, Mein-Lien related that her chest pain decreased. Muscle testing revealed that the functional strength of her subscapularis muscle returned to normal.

After addressing the compression of her heart from the back and from the encasing fascia within the chest cavity in the front, the doctor proceeded to the most likely provocative factor—the initial emotional trauma that led to these causes of the physical pain in Mei-Lien's heart. The doctor had her think about the moment she confronted her cousin about her betrayal, then preceded to test the subscapularis muscle closely connected to stress. It returned to its previously physiologically inhibited state while she maintained this mental picture. Her breathing became shallow and somewhat labored. Clearly, the deepest of the underlying causes still persisted.

The Applied Kinesiologist had Mei-Lien employ Therapy Localization by gently placing her hands on her forehead, as she had done repeatedly during the consultation. He tested the muscle again, and it became facilitated. Mei-Lien had unconsciously been utilizing this soothing technique by directly placing her fingers upon the mechanoreceptors on the skin over her forehead when thinking or talking about her stressful situation.

The doctor noticed the beneficial effects and proceeded to employ the more focused "stress receptor" AK modality known as Emotional Recall Technique (ERT). While this procedure is more commonly used to relieve gastrointestinal stress-related symptoms such as acid reflux, ulcers, gastritis, and even simple nausea, it was apparent that it would help Mei-Lien cope effectively with her painful memories.

The procedure consisted of the doctor lightly stimulating these receptors *while* Mei-Lien recalled the emotional trauma that sparked her physical complaints. She rested face up on the table with the doctor holding these points until he saw her breathing become calmer, signifying that the physiological response to this emotional stress had been alleviated. After having Mei-Lien clear her mind and take some deep breaths, the doctor again asked her to think about her cousin and the heartbreaking chain of events. This time there was no negative responses measured and no sign of respiratory distress. She experienced an immediate sense of feeling more refreshed and at peace than she had in a long time.

Mei-Lien had five additional treatments. Each time, she left with more energy and less pain. The doctor showed her how to stimulate the receptors herself when she felt stressed. The Applied Kinesiologist also gave Mei-Lien deep breathing exercises to open up her chest cavity and strengthening exercises for the lower trapezius and subscapularis muscles. When she returned for a follow-up treatment a month later, she was talkative and full of energy and smiles. Her chest pain and depression had finally lifted. With a new zest for life, she went on to make a unique blend of aromatherapy oils to help people suffering from stress.

* * *

Applied Kinesiology recognizes the reciprocal effects of the psychological and physiological dynamics on our total health. Since our neurological, muscular, and fascial systems carry electrical and chemical signals via neural impulses, any physical blockage in our body can affect our thoughts and emotions. For instance, NDS represents a *physiological* condition with *psychological* manifestations. Often, a traumatic emotional event can trigger a physiological imbalance that reinforces the problem.

Traditional medicine often overlooks the necessity of treating both aspects of the mind-body connection and focuses on either the psychological or the physical origins of a particular condition. Applied Kinesiology works in coordination with psychotherapy to aid in the treatment of many emotional disorders. Doctors using AK procedures can make physical corrections to help free patients from conditions often thought to be purely psychological in origin. These physical corrections can reduce internal stress and allow for a more clear and confident response to external circumstances, as well as help us to maintain control over ourselves and our lives.

16

SEXUAL DYSFUNCTION AND INFERTILITY

The reproductive system is a collection of internal and external organs, in both females and males, that is highly regulated by hormones. The hormones are produced by the ovaries and testes, or by other endocrine glands including the adrenal, thyroid, pituitary, hypothalamus, and pineal.

The male reproductive organs include the testes, urethra, vas deferens, prostate, and penis. The prostate gland is a walnut-sized structure that sits below the bladder and in front of the rectum. A tube called the urethra runs from the bladder through the center of the prostate to the penis to expel urine from the body. The prostate also secretes fluid that nourishes and protects the sperm made in the testicles. Another tube called the vas deferens carries sperm from the testes to the seminal vesicles, and, during ejaculation, the prostate squeezes this mixture of sperm and fluid through the urethra out of the penis as semen. The testes are carried in an external pouch called the scrotum, where they normally remain cooler than the temperature of the rest of the body to facilitate sperm production and vitality.

The female reproductive organs include the ovaries, fallopian tubes, uterus, cervix, and vagina. The ovaries produce an ovum (egg) that is released monthly to travel through the fallopian tubes to the uterus, where it can be fertilized by sperm that enters the cervix. Once fertilized, the ovum becomes a zygote and develops into a fetus within the uterus that is located in the middle of the pelvis. Natural birth occurs when the fetus is pushed through the vagina after nine months in the uterus. These internal organs prefer a warm environment for function and fertility, as demonstrated by the rise in a woman's core body temperature during ovulation to prepare the uterine lining for a possible pregnancy.

Common signs and symptoms of male and female reproductive system disorders include abdominal and pelvic pain, abnormal vaginal discharge, menstrual irregularities including heavy bleeding or severe pain with periods, burning and/or itchiness of genitals, pain or discomfort during sexual intercourse, ejaculatory or erectile dysfunction, and infertility—defined as the inability to conceive or the inability of male sperm to fertilize an ovum.

The physical conditions that can adversely affect the reproductive system include trauma, polycystic ovary syndrome (PCOS), prostatitis, endometriosis, sperm deficiencies, ovarian insufficiency, erectile dysfunction (ED), uterine fibroids, ejaculatory disorders, sexually transmitted diseases (STDs), pelvic inflammatory disease, benign prostatic hypertrophy (BPH), and various cancers such as ovarian, penile, breast, prostate, cervical, and testicular.

Less commonly known, but equally important conditions, are the various *functional issues* that can affect your reproductive system. Like all the systems in the body, the reproductive system is integrated into the neuro-muscular-organ complex. As a result, the position or proper movement of the system that encases the organs of reproduction is vital to their healthy function. Any disruption in the delicate balance of these systems can impact the complex processes of reproduction. For instance, if the pelvis is misaligned and constricted, the organs contained within the pelvic area such as the ovaries, uterus, prostate, bowels, and bladder and their controlling neural innervation can also become compromised—creating dysfunction.

The first step in the functional approach to the treatment of non-pathological sexual dysfunction and infertility is to restore normalcy to the structures that contain and control the sex organs. This is successfully accomplished by realigning the pelvic bones and restoring full motion to the sacroiliac and pubic joint, as well as the rest of the spinal and cranial segments. These realignments allow optimal function of the pelvic muscles while restoring full neural innervation to the related organs of the reproductive system.

Entrapment of the pelvic nerves, such as the *pudendal nerve* and other nerves coming from the lower and mid-back area, as well as the cranial bones of the skull, can affect your sexual organs and lead to infertility and sexual dysfunction. Functional muscle testing allows your Applied Kinesiologist to examine you for pelvic, endocrine, and neural dysfunctions—which are readily reversible in most cases. Applied Kinesiology therapies have proven to be very successful in restoring normal function to men and women with non-pathological sexual dysfunction and infertility issues.

Sexual dysfunction refers to a problem occurring during any phase of the *sexual response cycle* that prevents an individual or couple from experiencing physical and emotional satisfaction from sexual activity. The sexual response cycle generally includes desire, excitement, orgasm, and resolution where the body slowly returns to its normal level of functioning, accompanied by a sense of well-being. This condition can impact the reproductive process as well.

Sexual dysfunction falls into three basic categories: desire disorders, excitement disorders, and orgasm disorders. The principal desire disorder in both men and women is hypoactive sexual desire disorder. This condition is characterized by a general lack of sexual desire or interest in having sex. Excitement disorders involve the inability to become physically aroused during sexual activity. In men, it is characterized by erectile dysfunction. In women, it can involve a lack of lubrication in the vagina. Orgasmic disorders involve an inability to achieve orgasm or reaching a physical climax too early in the sexual process, such as in premature ejaculation in men which can affect satisfaction in both partners.

These conditions can occur at any age after maturity, though it is more common in individuals over the age of forty and generally related to hormonal and physiological changes often associated with aging and a corresponding decline in overall health. In the United States, female sexual dysfunction has been estimated to affect over 40% of women in the general population.[54] In the

United States, almost 50% of men over 40 report some degree of sexual dysfunction.[55]

INFERTILITY AND IMPAIRED FECUNDITY

Pregnancy is the result of a complex set of processes that include a woman releasing an egg from one of her ovaries (ovulation), a man's sperm joining with the egg along the way (fertilization), the fertilized egg going through a fallopian tube toward the uterus (womb), and the fertilized egg attaching to the inside of the womb (implantation). Infertility can arise from a problem with any of these steps.

Clinically, infertility is defined as the inability to get pregnant after one year or longer of unprotected intercourse. Approximately 12-15% of married couples have trouble getting pregnant.[55] Statistics reveal that 1/3 of infertility is attributed to the female; 1/3 to the male; and 1/3 is due to a combination of problems in both partners.[56]

Impaired fecundity is the term used for a woman who may be experiencing difficulty sustaining her pregnancy to full or near full term. The United States Census Bureau has reported a reduction in population growth due to an increase in both infertility and impaired fecundity. At the current rate of increase of these two conditions, they are projecting that nearly one-third of the female population will have impaired fecundity or infertility.

Factors that can negatively affect a woman's ability to become pregnant or to carry to full term include smoking, age, poor nutrition, eating disorders, alcohol intake, sexually transmitted diseases (STDs), hormonal imbalance, drug use, stress, depression, menstrual irregularity, exposure to environmental toxins, and certain pathological conditions affecting the reproduction organs such as polycystic ovarian syndrome or endometriosis. Treatments for infertility and impaired fecundity include stimulating ovulation with fertility drugs, intrauterine insemination (the insertion of healthy sperm directly into the uterus), and *in vitro* fertilization, wherein an egg is fertilized with a sperm outside of the uterus then inserted into the uterus. In cases of impaired fecundity, sustained bed rest is prescribed to facilitate carrying to full term during pregnancy.

The principal conditions related to male infertility include issues with sexual function, such as erectile dysfunction, ejaculatory disorders, lowered sperm count or motility, and conditions causing painful intercourse, such as Peyronie's disease (where fibrous scar tissue leads to a significantly curved penis and painful erections).

Factors affecting male fertility include use of alcohol, tobacco or other drugs; hernia surgery; diabetes; poor nutrition; STDs; severe mumps infection after puberty; low testosterone; blockage of sperm most commonly from a varicocele (an enlarged vein in testicle); and retrograde ejaculation (where semen enters the bladder instead of exiting out of the body through the penis). Environmental causes include overexposure to industrial chemicals, heavy metals, and radiation; overheating the testicles from hot tubs and saunas; wearing tight clothing; prolonged sitting; and working with a laptop computer on one's lap. These can increase the temperature of the scrotum and reduce sperm production. Current treatments for non-pathological causes of male infertility include lifestyle changes such as avoiding the above causative factors, adopting a sensible diet and exercise program, stopping certain medications and other drugs, and taking other medications to try to improve sperm production and quality.

In addition to these factors, there are numerous *functional* problems that many people are unaware of that can cause sexual dysfunction or infertility which often manifest as other seemingly unrelated health conditions.

* * *

MARY, 42, was happy being a wife, home manager, and part-time freelance photographer. She and her husband, a contractor, traveled, frequented sporting events, and enjoyed each other's company. After ten years of marriage, they decided to start a family. Mary was thirty-eight and had stopped her birth control pills, but after several months she began experiencing some bloating, mood swings, and headaches. She reasoned that these symptoms were due to her return to her natural hormone levels and just accepted it.

However, after nearly two years, they were having no luck getting pregnant. She consulted with her gynecologist, who suggested that they see a fertility specialist. She and her husband both took various tests to pinpoint any physical issues that might be affecting their fertility. The results were all negative, indicating that there was no apparent physical problem. The specialist suggested a range of treatment options starting with fertility drugs and various procedures, such as artificial or *in vitro* fertilization.

They decided to start with fertility drugs. They worked on two occasions, but both times Mary could not carry to full term. After her second miscarriage, Mary began experiencing excruciating low back pain. It seemed that the infertility condition had been complicated by something also causing impaired fecundity. The entire process was depressing and stressful, which contributed to her back problems.

Their fertility doctor thought that her back pain was related to the stress of their challenges to getting and remaining pregnant. He suggested that she see a chiropractor to relieve her symptoms. Mary had been to a chiropractic doctor in the past for some minor issues relating to her knee, so she made an appointment. Her doctor had become certified in AK since she last visited him.

After completing the patient profile, Mary and her husband went into the consultation room. During the consultation, the doctor inquired about the history of her recent back pain. When Mary described the years of trying to get pregnant, fertility treatments, and the two miscarriages, she began crying about their almost four years of failure and frustration. While her husband consoled her, the doctor could see that Mary was unable to twist her back to the right and had to lift her pelvis off the chair to hug him back.

When the doctor questioned about her pain in that area, Mary mentioned that she had sharp pain since her second miscarriage, and before that, she felt slight numbness in the area. She shared the additional information that, occasionally, sexual intercourse would create some pain in the pubic and groin region as well.

Postural Analysis revealed a pronounced swayback, a condition in which the lower spine curves inward and forces the pelvis forward along with a twisting of the pelvis. Her pain symptoms and posture mimicked those related to pelvic girdle pain (PGP), with pain in the sacroiliac joints and symphysis pubis joint in the front, which often occurs in pregnant women. Gait Analysis revealed that Mary walked as if she was twisting to one side; her right leg stepped out from the midline and veering out to the right.

During the examination, the doctor found that her pelvis was misaligned. She had a misalignment of her sacroiliac joint where the pelvic bone (ilium) meets the tailbone (sacrum), as well as of the pubic symphysis joint where the pubic bones meet. Applied Kinesiological FMT revealed a physiological inhibition of her right gluteus maximus, hamstrings, and adductor (groin) muscles, as well as tightness of her right piriformis muscle—all of which would lead to the twisting of her pelvis and splaying of her right leg.

The doctor asked her about any exercises that she routinely did. Mary explained that she didn't exercise, but that she often got into awkward positions including twisting, doing partial splits, and squatting down low to the ground while photographing weddings or catching animals in nature. She always carried her camera gear on her left side and twisted to the left frequently to change lenses or cameras. The doctor concluded that these positions caused her to habitually torque her pelvis, which had gradually subluxated her joints and lower spine.

The doctor diagnosed her with pelvic girdle pain (PGP) secondary to misalignment of the right sacroiliac joint in her back, her symphysis pubic joint in the front, and a sprained pelvis—all resulting in entrapment of various pelvic nerves and organ dysfunction.

The abnormal movement of the pelvic joints affected the neural control of the muscles of the pelvis as well as the sexual and reproductive organs, including the uterus and vagina. This dysfunction could have been a significant factor for her occasionally painful intercourse, fertility issues, and subsequent miscarriages. Mary was unsure of what to make of this, so the doctor put it another way: "If your pelvis is twisted, the organs contained within the pelvic girdle can become *twisted* and cease to function properly."

On top of the other pelvic functional problems, Mary developed Piriformis Syndrome, or what AK doctors call Sprained Pelvis Syndrome. In this condition, the piriformis muscle often becomes tight and can affect the nerves to the gluteus medius (superior gluteal nerve), gluteus maximus (inferior gluteal nerve), the hamstrings (sciatic nerve), and the sex organs via the pudendal nerve which is also very close to the piriformis muscle.

The *pudendal nerve* arises from what is called the sacral plexus. It is made of the second, third and fourth nerve roots (known as S2, S3, S4). This nerve must traverse through two openings known as the greater sciatic foramen and the lesser sciatic foramen. This nerve travels very close to the piriformis muscle. If there is a misalignment of the sacrum (through which the nerves travel) or the pelvis in general due to a Sprained Pelvis Syndrome, this misalignment can affect the pudendal nerve, other sacral nerves essential for proper functioning of the reproductive organs (such as the pelvic splanchnic nerves which also arise from S2, S3, S4), and the delicate positioning of the organs themselves.

When the doctor placed a sacroiliac support belt over her pelvis and tested the gluteus, hamstring, and piriformis muscles, they returned to normal physiological function. Mary felt relief from her back pain as well. This revealed that the inhibition of the gluteus maximus and hamstrings muscles were due to a peripheral entrapment of the inferior gluteal nerve and sciatic nerve, respectively. With the wearing of the belt, the spasm of the piriformis muscle released, indicating that its tightness was secondary to the sprain of the pelvis. The doctor said that the treatment would begin by facilitating the muscles controlled by these nerves. Once they were functioning properly, there was a good chance that Mary's reproductive organs would no longer be impacted.

The doctor removed the supportive belt and had Mary lie on the examination table on her side. He performed a precise chiropractic adjustment to the sacroiliac joint between the sacral and iliac bone of the pelvis. He then had Mary lie face up and squeeze a rolled-up towel between her knees. This caused an audible click from her groin area, indicating a successful realignment of her pubic bones. The realignment of the pubic symphysis and sacroiliac joint would relieve the severe PGP (pelvic girdle pain) that she was experiencing. It also restored normal function to the adductor muscle that attached to the pubic bone.

Afterward, the doctor had Mary lie face down, and he placed soft wedges known as Sacro-Occipital Technique (SOT) blocks beneath her pelvis. This technique is used to help remove the tension in the pelvic region due to the chronic stress of twisting. This condition is common in people who habitually twist predominately in one way—as Mary did to change lenses or cameras. Other common scenarios include people sitting at a desk that twist in one direction to work, those who habitually cross one leg over the other, playing twisting sports like golf, or carrying a handbag over one shoulder. These are all susceptible to developing this torqueing condition of the pelvic girdle.

Mary felt immediate relief after the blocks were removed. The doctor recommended that she wear the belt as much as possible for the next month to help stabilize the bones and muscles of the region and ensure the continual release of pressure on the pelvic nerves and organs.

Mary required 12 treatments in total to restore optimal physiological function to the muscles, bones, nerves and reproductive organs of her pelvis. The doctor instructed her to carry her camera gear on alternate sides of her body equally to eliminate her twisting to the same side and to temporarily limit her photo jobs to those that did not require awkward positions. Within two months of the initial visit, Mary's back pain and pelvic pain had disappeared completely. Soon after, she became pregnant without the use of fertility drugs. She visited the Applied Kinesiologist once a month to make sure that her pelvis was in proper alignment during the pregnancy. She and her husband were overjoyed to welcome their healthy baby boy.

* * *

VIVIAN, 31, and her husband had been trying to conceive for at least three years with no luck. They had been married for six years. Vivian was the office manager for her husband's dermatology practice. Together, they had firmly established his practice and, as they had planned, they were now ready for parenthood. After several years without success, they went for fertility tests—all of which turned out to be negative. Nothing obvious seemed to be preventing them from getting pregnant, and they were frustrated. However, one factor seemed to be consistent: Vivian's menstrual cycles were inconsistent. She had experienced this condition most of her adult life.

Also, she had trouble falling asleep and sleeping through the night without waking up numerous times. She was fatigued throughout most of every day and never felt like she ever really slept at night or ever fully woke up in the morning. The fertility specialist felt that the irregular menses and interrupted sleep patterns may be the cause of her infertility and suggested drugs to balance her hormones and help with her sleep. The next step would be fertility specific medications.

Vivian had experienced bad reactions with hormonal drugs over the years. When she had tried birth control pills to regulate her periods, she encountered severe physical and emotional symptoms. She and her husband decided to try to get her sleep cycles in order first to see if that would help. She previously tried over-the-counter sleeping pills, which helped but made her feel even more sluggish than usual the next day. She resorted to the natural supplement melatonin, which initially worked well to help her sleep; unfortunately, she eventually developed a tolerance, and it no longer had the desired effect.

Unsure about what to do next, they decided to see a holistic doctor, who specialized in AK and had an office in the same building as her husband's practice, before trying any prescription drugs. Their receptionist had gone to this doctor for several health complaints and said that he always seemed to find a solution to her problems.

During the consultation, the doctor immediately noticed that Vivian looked somewhat pale and had dark rings under her eyes. In studying the detailed patient profile, the doctor also noticed a pattern with Vivian's complaints. Most had to do with sleep and menstrual cycles, which indicated an issue with her circadian rhythms. Each person has a particular sensitivity to daily, monthly, and seasonal cycles. Vivian's cycles were seriously disrupted daily by lack of sleep. Monthly chronic menstrual irregularities were evident, wavering between twenty-one to forty days apart. She also stated that she suffered from seasonal depression, also known as seasonal affective disorder (SAD), a condition linked to changes in light throughout the year.

Whenever a person has a problem with their circadian cycles, it often indicates some issue relating to pineal gland function. The pineal gland is located between the two cerebral hemispheres of the brain. It is shaped like a small pine cone, which is how it got its name. Your pineal gland is an endocrine gland that has no direct connection to your central nervous system; rather, it is controlled by environmental lighting or photoperiodism that are conveyed through the optic nerves with indirect signals from the sympathetic nerves (superior cervical ganglia).

Therefore, your pineal gland is similar to your adrenal medulla in that it converts signals from your sympathetic nervous system to secrete and release hormones, in this case, melatonin. Melatonin has long been recognized for its effects on sleep-wake and menstrual cycles. It is essential for the regulation of reproductive cycles as well. Synthesis and secretion of melatonin are dramatically affected by light exposure to the eyes. Light exposure to the retina of your eye is relayed to the hypothalamus gland, which in turn sends signals to your spinal cord, where the nerves in your neck (superior cervical ganglia) send the information back to the pineal gland. Concentrations of melatonin are low during the daylight hours and increase to a peak during the night.

Using these facts, Applied Kinesiologists have found a physiological screening procedure to measure the functional ability of your pineal gland. While AK research has not found the pineal gland to be related to any one specific muscle, your doctor can functionally test other muscles, most commonly certain muscles empirically found to be related to the endocrine system; then, by darkening the room or covering your face from sensing light, he or she can measure any physiological disruption of these muscles. If this AK procedure, known as the Pineal Light Challenge, reveals inhibition of any of these endocrine-related muscles, it indicates a functional problem with your pineal gland.

In Vivian's case, every muscle the doctor tested recorded physiological inhibition after the room was darkened. Vivian and her husband were shocked. She innately grasped the significance of these findings. It clearly demonstrated why Vivian never felt refreshed after sleeping. She was not neurophysiologically recharging herself when she slept, probably due to some dysfunction of the pineal gland. This condition could be a major factor in her inability to conceive.

The examination continued with the doctor inspecting her cranial bones and jaw muscles; they were severely tight and restricted. When the doctor spread apart specific cranial bones, she no longer experienced physiological inhibition to her muscles in darkness—indicating that the resulting pressure within the skull was interfering with the function of her pineal gland.

Zinc is a key element in pineal gland health and an important regulator of melatonin synthesis. In fact, studies have suggested that the highest concentration of this vital mineral in women is found in the pineal gland. The doctor had Vivian do a taste test with a high-quality zinc supplement and found her deficient in this mineral.

The doctor diagnosed her with a physiological dysfunction of her pineal gland. The treatment involved a procedure known as The Pineal Technique. It involves gentle cranial manipulation to the parietal, sphenoid, maxillary, and mandibular bones to release any pressure and neural dysfunction of the gland. In addition to the cranial treatment, Vivian was given a high-quality zinc supplement and was instructed to include foods rich in zinc. She was also advised to eat foods high in the amino acid tryptophan every day such as turkey, chicken, tuna, shrimp, cheese, and organic eggs. She was taught to habitually have complex carbohydrate foods in her evening meal such as pasta, sweet potatoes, peas, brown or black rice. Research has shown that complex carbohydrates increase the transportation of tryptophan across the blood-brain barrier, which can help increase your brain's levels of the important neurotransmitters and hormones—serotonin and melatonin.

The Applied Kinesiologist also encouraged Vivian to expose her eyes to more natural outdoor light. She was to get more sunlight whenever possible, especially in the morning—allowing sunlight to shine directly upon her forehead for a few minutes. She initially resisted and stated that she was afraid of wrinkles and had not let the sun touch her face in over 10 years. The doctor explained that her "natural light deficiency" could be a contributing factor and assured her that 10 minutes of direct morning sunlight would be fine for her skin and important for her pineal health and fertility. She agreed. Vivian also adopted a "no screen" policy at night at least two hours before bed, since the artificial blue light from television, computers, and cell phones have been shown to disrupt melatonin secretion and sleep regulation. She was also instructed to no longer leave a nightlight on in the bedroom.

Vivian returned in three days and said that she was already sleeping more deeply and feeling better in the morning. The doctor continued to treat her with The Pineal Technique during this treatment session and four subsequent visits—each time needing to correct fewer cranial and jaw restrictions.

Within three months, Vivian reported that she was sleeping much better, and, for the first time in her life, she had predictable menstrual periods. Her circadian rhythms were finally on track, and she had little trouble getting pregnant shortly thereafter.

Erectile Dysfunction

Erectile dysfunction (ED), or male impotence, is a condition in which a man has consistent problems achieving and/or maintaining an erection. ED is among the most common disorders of male sexual health. This condition is reported in 40% of men after 40 and increases to nearly 70% in men at age 70.[57] Symptoms of ED include an inability to achieve an erection, erections that are too soft for penetration during sexual intercourse, and inability to maintain an erection long enough to engage in sexual intercourse. In the past, erectile function was commonly believed to be predominately a marker for cardiovascular dysfunction in older men. However, new research has shown that there are a variety of causes for this condition which are not necessarily heart-related and that 25% of men seeking help for ED were under the age of 40.

An erection occurs when blood fills the two chambers in the penis. These individual chambers are called the corpus cavernosa. When they fill with blood, they cause the penis to stiffen and expand. This hardening process is triggered and maintained by neural impulses from the brain and genital nerves in the lower back. Anything that blocks these *nerve impulses* or restricts blood flow to the penis can result in erectile dysfunction.

Penile erection is also dependent on nitric oxide. Nitric oxide is an important chemical that helps to maintain blood vessel health and regulate blood pressure. It is produced in the lining of blood vessels and helps to dilate them. Many drugs such as Viagra, Levitra, and Cialis help to increase the production of nitric oxide to dilate the arteries to increase blood flow and are used to achieve stronger erections. Nitric oxide levels can be increased naturally as well from foods containing high levels of the amino acids, citrulline, and arginine, such as walnuts, beets, rhubarbs, dark, leafy green vegetables like spinach and arugula, garlic, watermelon, turkey, grass-fed beef, seafood, and dark chocolate. Exercise also increases your nitric oxide levels as does breathing in through your nose, since nitric oxide is also produced within the paranasal sinuses. Additionally, nasal nitric oxide is known to be increased up to 20-fold by strong humming compared with quiet expiration—with potential beneficial effects throughout the body.

Another factor in ED is a deficiency in testosterone. It is a hormone important for male sexual characteristics, muscle development and maintenance, red blood cells, bone growth, overall health, and sexual function. This hormone is essential to libido and in preventing sexual desire disorders. Research has shown that nearly 25% of men over 30 years old experience lower levels of testosterone,[58] which can also lead to erectile dysfunction.

There are many systemic problems and lifestyle habits that can lead to erectile dysfunction. Some factors that can create circulatory and nerve problems resulting in ED include diabetes, cardiovascular and kidney disease, smoking, excessive alcohol consumption, inactivity, obesity, and drug use. Also, medications for blood pressure, depression, and anxiety often have side effects that can cause the inability to get an erection. Occasionally, surgical treatments for prostate or bladder conditions can damage the nerves to the penis and result in ED. While most cases of ED have a physical cause, there are psychological factors that can contribute to ED as well, including depression, stress, poor self-esteem, and performance anxiety about sex.

Doctors will perform standard exams which often include blood and urine tests to uncover if an underlying condition, adverse reaction to medication, or lifestyle choices are causing the problem. If none are found, the doctor will probably prescribe an oral medication to increase blood flow to the penis. In some cases, the drugs will be injected directly into the penis or by inserting a pellet inside of the shaft. If the condition is serious enough, some doctors will prescribe a vacuum device (pump) which is placed over the penis to draw the blood into the chambers to create an erection before intercourse. An elastic band is worn around the base of the penis to maintain the erection during sex.

In more serious cases, surgery might be indicated, such as in the case of a blockage in an artery or vein that prevents sufficient blood flow into the penis. This condition most often occurs as a result of a groin injury. If a penile implant is recommended, two hollow tubes are inserted into the carpi cavernosa and inflated with air with a hand pump when an erection is desired. After intercourse, the air is released.

As discussed, there are many possible causes of erectile dysfunction. However, the most common cause, in otherwise healthy individuals, is biomechanical or structural. One such structural cause of ED is what is called a varicocele. A varicocele is a dilatation of the pampiniform venous plexus and the internal spermatic vein. Varicocele is a well-recognized cause of decreased testicular function and can create male fertility problems with lower testosterone and sperm production as well as a diminished sex drive. It occurs in approximately 15%-20% of all males and in 40% of infertile males.[59] It often occurs due to increased pressure on the testicular vein from compression of the renal vein. Surgery might be indicated if a blockage in an artery or vein impeding blood flow is found. A high-resolution color-flow Doppler ultrasonography is the diagnostic method of choice in patients with suspected varicocele.

Another structural problem that causes sexual dysfunction in men has to do with the positional alignment of the pelvis. A bony misalignment of the lumbar and pelvic bones can affect erectile function. The penis is innervated by a complex system of somatic and autonomic nerve fibers that run through the spinal vertebrae which control sensory and motor function necessary for sexual response. The dorsal nerve branches off from the *pudendal nerve* and provides impulses to the penis. Tactile stimulation is transmitted back to the spinal cord which, in turn, increases blood flow to initiate the erection response. The dorsal nerve also plays a role in maintaining an erection and the discharge of ejaculatory fluid during orgasm. Inhibition to these nerves, through misalignment of the sacrum and pelvis, can lead to ED.

* * *

ELI, 31, started experiencing ejaculatory and later erectile dysfunction when he was twenty-seven. He was generally healthy and enjoyed a rigorous routine of gym workouts and weightlifting. On and off over the years, he suffered from low back pain, often linked to heavy weight lifting, but just accepted it as part of the process. After he had been married for a few years, he and his wife were ready to start a family. One day at the gym, he experienced sharp low back pain centered in the left buttocks, tail bone, and in the perineal (the area between the rectum and scrotum). Soon after, he began to experience problems in getting an erection. He always had enjoyed a fulfilling sexual life, and he was understandably concerned by this new development.

Eli went to see a urologist, who prescribed 5 mg of Cialis each day. Not experiencing any change, he tried Viagra at a higher dose—still no results. He also suffered from constipation and deep pain during bowel movements. He was referred to a proctologist, who took a litany of tests to determine whether there was any kind of pathological problem or obstruction, such as a tumor. They found that he had two conditions: prostatitis, or inflammation of the prostate gland, and *outlet dysfunction constipation*, a condition that causes the anal sphincter muscle to contract instead of relax during defecation. Eli took a series of medications, but nothing relieved his conditions.

Since medications didn't seem to be helping, one of his doctors suggested that because all of these problems seemed to have started after his lower back injury, he try chiropractic or osteopathic treatments. The doctor suggested that spinal manipulation and realignment could be successful in restoring normal movement to the lumbar and pelvic spinal bones, relieve the lower back pain, and, perhaps, help with his sexual dysfunction and constipation. He referred him to a doctor who was also a specialist in AK.

During the initial visit, Eli shared that he was deeply upset and frustrated about his condition and could not understand why every specialist he consulted could not come up with a solution to his problems. The doctor stated that since no one could find a pathological reason for his ED, the chances were good that the reason was *functional* in nature, as his doctor suggested, and could be cured.

Reading the patient forms and medical records, the doctor saw that Eli had a previous history of inguinal hernias on both sides of his lower abdomen, most likely due to his strenuous workout routine. He had already undergone surgery that fixed the problem and continued his regimen of lifting until his most recent injury. The Applied Kinesiologist strongly suspected that the sacral nerves which affect the rectum, pelvic muscles, and the penis were suffering from some kind of neural inhibition due to the accident at the gym.

Postural Analysis revealed Eli had an extreme inward curve of the spine, also known as a swayback. In other words, from the side view, he appeared to be sticking his buttocks out and looked like he was arching backward. Gait Analysis revealed that Eli walked with both legs splaying outwards to such a degree that he looked like he was imitating the famous walk of the actor Charlie Chaplin.

AK functional muscle testing revealed a physiological inhibition of both of his gluteus maximus muscles and tightness of both of his piriformis muscles, which would lead to the sway- back and splaying of his feet. Additional FMT uncovered a bilateral physiological inhibition of his hip flexor and lumbar spine stabilizing muscles (psoas), as well as the muscles that connect the ribcage with the pelvis (quadratus lumborum). Palpation of his spine revealed jamming of his upper lumbar spinal bones; functional muscle testing confirmed these findings.

The doctor surmised that Eli's weight lifting was the most likely cause for all of these issues. The doctor asked Eli to demonstrate his weight lifting technique in the office. As suspected, the doctor saw that Eli was not using the proper form—that was the most likely reason for the sharp pain caused by an anterior subluxation of his sacrum and jamming (facet imbrication) of his upper lumbar spinal vertebrae.

The doctor explained that years of improper technique and the recent weight lifting accident caused the muscles in his low back to seize up and the vertebrae to compress, which affected the nerves responsible for sexual performance.

Neurologically, the sympathetic nerves in the spinal column emitting from between the lower thoracic and upper lumbar (T11-L2) control *ejaculation* and the nerves exiting the sacrum (S2-S4) control penile *erection*. These nerves, including the pudendal nerve, were pressured by the vertebral misalignments, thereby preventing them from performing their neural signaling function.

The doctor explained that the pudendal nerve arises from what is called the sacral plexus. It is made of the second, third, and fourth nerve roots (known as S2, S3, S4). The pudendal nerve carries sensations from the penis and is responsible for the afferent (feeling) component of an erection, and it also supplies motor function to the anal sphincter. Thus, if the pudendal nerve is affected, it can create both erectile dysfunction and constipation.

The doctor diagnosed Eli as suffering from entrapment of the pudendal nerve. AK doctors find this condition to be a frequent cause of ED. The good news was that these conditions were all reversible but would require several different modes of treatment. The doctor began by performing precise adjustments to the T12, L1 and L2 spinal vertebrae, as well as employing the AK muscle manipulation techniques of Spindle Cell Restoration to both of Eli's psoas and *fascial release* to his quadratus lumborum muscles. Eli felt immediate relief of his sharp low back pain and was already feeling more comfortable.

Then the AK practitioner used a sacrotuberous ligament release technique (also called Logan Basic Technique) to free up the pudendal nerve. After administering this specialized procedure, he proceeded to implement a highly specific adjustment maneuver, known as "segmental drop adjusting" (sometimes called Thompson

Technique), wherein normal motion is restored to the sacrum to re-establish optimal structural and neural function to the pelvis and sex glands. It would also relieve his constipation and prostatitis.

The doctor instructed Eli to stop weightlifting for the duration of his treatments. He further advised him to add psyllium husks to his diet to keep the colon clear and pumpkin seeds for their high levels of zinc, fiber, and phytosterols, which have been shown to help with prostate health.

Eli required 10 visits in total to stabilize the thoracolumbar spine, sacral bone, and pelvic muscles. The Applied Kinesiologist had him wear a sacroiliac belt to expedite the healing of the pelvis. He referred him to a physical therapist who gave Eli exercises to help with the pelvic diaphragm, gluteus maximus, and piriformis muscles; as well as instructed him to engage in more weight *training* and less weight *lifting*. Along with being in excellent shape, Eli no longer suffered from constipation or back pain and, best of all, had no erectile dysfunction issues. He and his wife have a two-year-old daughter and are expecting another child.

* * *

The ability to engage in sexual activity, to become pregnant, and to give birth are basic human activities that are rife with potential difficulties including sexual dysfunction, infertility, and impaired fecundity. While medical procedures and pharmaceuticals abound to help men and women overcome these problems, lead a fulfilling sex life, and achieve their parenting dream; these traditional medical treatments are often not effective. In many cases, they overlook the functional source of the conditions.

Applied Kinesiology offers natural solutions for these conditions. Misalignments of the bones that make up the pelvic girdle can create physical and physiological barriers impeding sexual function, as well as fertility and pregnancy-related issues. Specific muscle manipulations, precise spinal, pelvic, and cranial bone adjustments, along with dietary and lifestyle modifications can enhance neural and physiological factors to restore sexual function and facilitate fertility.

17

YOUR JOURNEY TO HEALTH

Hippocrates, known as the Father of Modern Medicine, said more than 2,000 years ago, "It is more important to know what sort of person has a disease than to know what sort of disease a person has."

Applied Kinesiology is founded on this credo. It is a holistic healing discipline dedicated to finding the unique source of each individual's physiological dysfunction and tailoring the best course of treatment for that particular *person* instead of a generic protocol for the condition. For instance, 10 people can present to an AK practitioner with the same low back pain symptoms. Yet, upon examination, the AK doctor might find that the actual source of their pain is different in each case. Each person will then require a unique treatment.

Applied Kinesiology's functional approach to healing relies upon the idea that every system in the body: bones, muscles, nerves and neural connections, glands, organs, cardiovascular, respiratory and fascia work cohesively. Any imbalance in the functionality of any part within these systems affects the entire body and can cause dysfunction and pain. Since dysfunction usually precedes or accompanies pain, AK's unique diagnostic technique of FMT can effectively uncover impairment within these integrated systems.

Pain is a powerful message from your body that there is some imbalance in those systems. Applied Kinesiology helps to decipher that message to help restore the balance or homeostasis of the body. True healing comes from within, and the job of the doctor is to remove any impediments to this healing to restore good health. The body is an amazing set of checks and balances. It knows how to heal itself if allowed to do so. Applied Kinesiology facilitates this process. Once you and your AK doctor correct the root cause of the problem, you will enjoy excellent health along with a greater sense of well-being and freedom from pain.

The doctor/patient relationship is the cornerstone of AK. Since there is a myriad of factors that can contribute to any dysfunction in the body, an AK specialist needs to get a full profile of a person before he or she can begin a proper examination. In addition to any symptoms related to the current condition, a patient's lifestyle, past injuries, sources of stress, and dietary habits are all important. The AK doctor spends a considerable amount of time gathering this information to gain a fuller understanding of the total person. Often, there are aspects of a person's experiences that point to the underlying nature of the condition. They can be as simple as the way you stand, sit, walk, hold your hands or turn your head. Others might involve pain or the inability to perform activities that were easily done before the complaint. These signals are pieces in the puzzle of your health that the Applied Kinesiologist assembles to create a dedicated diagnosis and treatment plan. This problem-solving skill set is at the core of AK's functional approach—to find the missing pieces and determine where they fit into your total health picture.

Applied Kinesiology is an ever-evolving evaluation system and embraces a wide variety of therapeutic techniques and modalities without first resorting to prescription drugs or surgery. It encompasses chiropractic, osteopathic, muscle manipulations, cranial therapy, acupuncture, nutrition, and visualization techniques. Whatever healing discipline the doctor employs is only the means to the end of achieving the successful outcome for the individual patient. Applied Kinesiology is predominately a proactive health-directed discipline designed to treat patients to not only cure the source of their problems but to prevent them from recurring in the future.

Traditional medicine has many benefits. Principal among them are the many technical tests available to gather information. Applied Kinesiology uses much of the information from these diagnostic tests to help get to the cause of health problems. But as one doctor said, "Tests can't tell you how well a patient lifts his or her arms, or climbs stairs, or reads or speaks; nor can it indicate personality or intelligence or sense of humor. Only patients can do that. The interpretation of test results depends entirely on what we learn from the details of their stories, comparisons to other patients and our own intuition."

Applied Kinesiology does not replace traditional medicine. All medical professionals rely upon examination and other data to arrive at a diagnosis. However, AK adds to and enhances traditional medicine by its holistic, functional assessment involving observation, listening, and muscle testing to uncover the underlying source of the problem. This functional approach allows your AK doctor to solve the mystery of your health issues by following the clues your body offers. Like a modern-day Sherlock Holmes (whom, incidentally, Dr. Arthur Conan Doyle modeled after his medical school professor, Dr. Joseph Bell), your Applied Kinesiologist pursues the facts to find the real "culprit" causing your condition.

Because of AK's natural, noninvasive approach to healing, patients seek it out as an option after the expensive and often limited treatments offered by traditional medicine fail to give relief. Many well-meaning doctors simply follow the protocols associated with the symptoms of the generic problems without actually getting to the root cause of the condition itself.

For many patients whose conditions are not cured by these routine treatments, AK becomes a discipline of last resort. For others, AK's straightforward alternative perspective on helping the body heal itself seems to make more sense to them than the more traditional approach. One could rationalize that the more conservative interventions offered by AK might, in certain circumstances when there is not a critical illness present, be considered as a *first* resort before more invasive methods are employed. Regardless of the reason, AK can help you become and remain healthy to enjoy a life free from pain and full of energy.

The body is an incredible neurophysiological system of biomechanical, biochemical and psychological components integrated and functioning together. From our heartbeat to our neural impulses, our physical and physiological systems are never at rest and are always in motion. Like any other moving entity, it can malfunction. Applied Kinesiology finds the actual source of the malfunction and restores it to full functionality. Applied Kinesiology is the gateway through which you can begin your own journey to healing.

APPENDICES

APPENDIX I

ELIMINATE ALLERGIES WITH APPLIED KINESIOLOGY

According to the Centers for Disease Control and Prevention (CDC), allergies are the sixth leading cause of chronic illness in the United States with an annual cost in excess of $18 billion. More than 50 million Americans suffer from allergies.[60] The World Health Organization reports that allergic rhinitis, otherwise known as seasonal allergies or "hay fever," occurs in 10% – 30% of the global population.[61] In Europe, seasonal allergies are reported to incur an annual cost of over 3,000,000,000 Euros.[62] Worldwide, the prevalence of allergic diseases has continued to rise in industrialized nations for more than 50 years.

The definition of an allergy is an *abnormal, exaggerated,* or *misguided* reaction to foreign substances generally considered to be harmless (allergens). This overreaction to a harmless substance is often called a hypersensitivity reaction. Almost anything can cause this reaction. Some of the most common allergens include certain kinds of food, dust, and pollen, pet dander, wool, latex, and some drugs like penicillin.

Unlike many common ailments, allergies are caused by a dysfunction of your neuro-immunological system. This dysfunction causes the immune system to become oversensitive and "overreact" to common external stimuli such as foods, environmental particles (pollens, animal dander), and other irritants. It is unclear what initiates this inappropriate activation of the immune system to protect the body from these nontoxic allergens. It is known that the initiating "trigger" is the assortment of proteins specific to the chemical profile of allergens. This is obvious in organic substances such as peanuts, seafood, and pollen allergies. However, even allergic reactions to synthetic substances such as latex and penicillin are because these also contain proteins. Latex is manufactured from the Hevea brasiliensis tree, a type of rubber tree that contains protein, and penicillin is heavily comprised of protein as well.

When introduced into the body, these select substances are met with resistance by the immune system, and it responds by releasing immunoglobulin E (IgE) antibodies which stimulate the mast cells to produce histamine—a naturally occurring chemical designed to create an inflammatory response to outside stimuli. Histamine release increases the permeability of the capillaries to leukocytes, commonly known as white blood cells, and allows them to enter into the bloodstream to engage pathogens, in this case, the particular proteins of the allergens. This inappropriate production of histamine is what causes the majority of symptoms commonly experienced in an allergic reaction.

Responding to this histamine production, the endocrine system releases the powerful anti-inflammatory hormone cortisol from the adrenal glands. If the adrenal glands don't produce enough cortisol, the allergic reaction can be amplified. The combination of histamine release and insufficient anti-inflammatory adrenal hormones in people with allergies often cause the common symptoms such as sneezing, runny nose, nasal congestion, post-nasal drip, throat irritation, wheezing and shortness of breath, a persistent, dry cough, skin rashes, fatigue, joint pains, headaches, brain fog, depression, nausea and vomiting, and even death from a very severe allergic reaction known as an anaphylactic reaction.

An allergy is generally diagnosed on the basis of the history of the patient's symptoms. The most common tests for determining if you have allergies are skin prick tests, blood tests, and oral food challenges. In the skin prick test, the doctor or nurse will prick your skin and expose you to small amounts of the proteins found in a wide variety of potential allergens. If you are allergic to any one of them, you will probably develop a raised bump or a hive at the test location on the skin.

Blood tests are used to measure the levels of immunoglobulin antibodies in your bloodstream associated with allergic reactions. Common blood tests include radioallergosorbent test (RAST) and ImmunoCAP testing. The RAST test consists of a technician drawing blood from you and placing it in a test tube, where the suspected allergen will be added to observe how much of that allergen binds to the IgE in your blood. ImmunoCAP testing involves the detection of allergen proteins by their binding a cellulose polymer in a plastic reserve.

An oral food challenge (OFC) is a procedure in which a food is eaten slowly in gradually increasing amounts, under medical supervision, to accurately diagnose or rule out a specific allergy to that food. OFCs are usually performed when a careful patient history and other tests are inconclusive. The oral food challenge is considered a more definitive test than the skin prick test or blood tests because it will show whether the food actually triggers a reaction or produces symptoms when consumed by the patient.

Traditional medicine has not been able to effectively address what causes the body to have allergic reactions; therefore, patients become dependent upon life-long medication. Its treatments are geared solely to reduce symptoms with over-the-counter and prescription medications administered in a variety of ways—oral, nasal, eye drops, topical creams, and injections that attempt to diminish allergy symptoms after they occur. These various medications include antihistamines, decongestants, anticholinergic nasal sprays, steroid nasal sprays, eye drops, mast cell inhibitors, leukotriene inhibitors, and auto-injectors. Side effects such as dry mouth, dizziness, restlessness, blurred vision, confusion, stomach problems, vomiting, increased blood pressure, headache, earache, insomnia, nervousness, nausea, skin irritation, and burning can occur.

Allergy shots and oral immunotherapy are used by allergy specialists to reduce sensitivity in people with severe symptoms. Immunotherapy generally takes three to five years of injections or life-long oral consumption to desensitize the person to the antigen. Side effects include swelling and redness at the injection site; allergy symptoms, such as a stuffy nose and watery eyes; difficulty breathing; throat tightness; abdominal pain; nausea; vomiting; irregular heartbeat; dizziness; loss of consciousness; and rarely, death.

Lifestyle modifications are the most common way to avoid allergic attacks, once the specific allergy has been established. These include avoiding the known food or allergen in conjunction with attempts to allergy-proof your environment. In the case of airborne allergens, many people find that using dehumidifiers, air filters, and ionizers, as well as deep cleaning and vacuuming along with using dust mite mattress and pillow covers can be effective.

Applied Kinesiology has developed a unique way of physiologically stopping allergies by restoring balance to your endocrine and immune systems' *oversensitivity* to certain allergens. This exclusive treatment is called The Allergy Technique. It has proven to be universally effective in helping people with allergies.

The procedure draws upon AK's multidisciplinary approach to healing. First, your doctor will require the standard full patient profile, including a detailed history and consultation. This profile should include all previous tests and treatments for the specific allergy in question. After the initial consultation and Postural and Gait Analysis, the doctor will first correct any obvious physiological problems. As most patients will visit the AK specialist displaying symptoms, your doctor will use the diagnostic procedures of FMT and TL to isolate the specific imbalances in your neuro/immunological/endocrine system that are causing the allergic reaction. If the patient is not displaying allergic symptoms at the time of the office visit, the doctor can utilize functional muscle testing to simulate the physiological allergic response to find the allergen as well as the optimal therapeutic option.

These immune imbalances manifest in one or more energy meridians among the approximately 365 acupuncture points throughout the body. Each of these points is associated with a particular aspect of the immune/endocrine systems, and uncovering the precise point(s) allows the AK specialist to effectively treat the underlying dysfunction creating the problem.

Once the appropriate points are discovered, the doctor will employ the specialized AK procedure of rhythmic stimulation therapy to these points by a gentle tapping procedure, which influences the hypothalamic-pituitary-adrenal (HPA) axis that is adversely stimulated in cases of allergens and restores balance. Quite often, in a few minutes upon the completion of the treatment, there is a cessation of the allergic reaction along with an immediate diminution of the accompanying symptoms such as watery eyes, congestion, coughing, and any skin rashes.

The principle behind this dramatic response is based upon studies that have shown acupuncture points to have a high density of receptors which, when properly activated, stimulate the nervous system to prevent, dampen and/or completely stop allergic reactions by lowering serum IgE levels. The Allergy Technique modulates the body's response through this mechanoreceptor stimulation to lower IgE levels which, in turn, reduces histamine and restores balance to the entire system. Performing this procedure while the patient is experiencing *hypersensitivity* symptoms intensifies the therapeutic benefit—with the immediate response of the body returning to homeostasis as well as preventing future allergic reactions.

The Allergy Technique is unique to AK because it approaches and treats allergic reactions from a functional perspective to uncover the imbalance of an individual's neural, immune, and endocrine systems. Once restored, the body will no longer have a hypersensitivity (allergic) reaction and, as a result, won't need to rely upon pharmaceuticals or avoidance of the allergens.

The Allergy Technique does not claim to be a cure for everyone. However, in most cases, this revolutionary AK technique successfully relieves and eliminates most serious allergic reactions immediately and restores normalcy regarding your particular allergen. Some patients require future treatments to ensure these reactions do not reoccur; however, once the treatment regimen is successfully administered, the result is usually permanent.

Practitioners can incorporate The Allergy Technique into their practice by learning it here: www.charlesseminars.com or (800) 351-5450

APPENDIX II

HOW TO FIND AN APPLIED KINESIOLOGY PRACTITIONER

There are thousands of Applied Kinesiologists throughout the world. Some are medical professionals with primary training in traditional medicine or other healing disciplines. In Europe, the majority of Applied Kinesiologists are medical doctors, physical therapists, and dentists. The United Kingdom consists of predominately osteopaths, chiropractors, naturopaths and MDs. AK doctors in Russia are MDs and PhDs. Korea has an equal mix of chiropractic and medical doctors along with dentists. In the United States, Canada, New Zealand, Australia, and Japan most doctors who utilize AK are doctors of chiropractic.

When doing your research, you need to find the person with the background and training with whom you feel the most comfortable. Most people seek out AK specialists through referrals from family and friends.

However, there are specific guidelines that will help you find the right professional for your own particular condition. These include:

1. The practitioner needs to be fully trained by a certified teaching Diplomate in Applied Kinesiology.
2. Find a practitioner who has experience treating people with your condition as you understand it from your symptoms

and information you received from other doctors, including medical specialists.

3. Since AK treatment usually involves multiple office visits and periodic follow-ups, you may need to take into consideration issues of proximity in your choice of a practitioner.

To find an Applied Kinesiologist in your area go to:

1. The International College of Applied Kinesiology: www.icak.com
2. The International College of Applied Kinesiology® USA: www.icakusa.com
3. Charles Seminars: www.charlesseminars.com

APPENDIX III

SAMPLE PATIENT QUESTIONNAIRE

An Applied Kinesiologist looks for clues to find the underlying cause of your health problems by gathering as much information as possible regarding a patient's past conditions to shed light on the present one.

A detailed patient profile is the essential first step in getting a complete picture of your overall well-being and allows for a full assessment of why you are currently experiencing health problems. Applied Kinesiology doctors use different patient profiles customized to their individual practices to serve their patients best. One commonality is that they will incorporate questions to assess the integrity of the different systems including your autonomic nervous system, cardiovascular system, respiratory system, digestive system, endocrine system, immune system, and musculoskeletal system.

Here is a sample patient questionnaire used by many Applied Kinesiologists:

A) Patients are asked to explain in detail the reason for their appointment
B) Date of illness/injury or how long they have not been feeling well
C) List their five main complaints in order of their severity

D) Describe the circumstances of each
E) List all doctors seen for the main condition and any other conditions
F) List all diagnoses given by these doctors
G) List any medication currently taking or previously taken
H) List any vitamin, mineral, and herbal supplements currently taking
I) List any allergies
J) List any recent surgeries
K) List any other previous surgeries or medical procedures
L) List childhood and family health history

A line drawing of a person is supplied for the patient to circle the location and to indicate the level of pain they are experiencing from 0 (no pain) to 10 (severe pain). Letters to describe the nature of the complaint are often used, such as A for achy, D for dull, B for burning, S for sharp, ST for stabbing, N for numbness, and PN for pins & needles.

A comprehensive checklist that creates a total picture of the kinds of issues that may impact the condition are as follows:

1. Feel cold often
2. Spicy foods upset stomach
3. Difficulty swallowing
4. Dry eyes, nose or mouth.
5. Heart rate elevates after eating
6. Difficulty relaxing
7. Cuts heal slowly
8. Gag easily
9. Startle easily
10. Cold or clammy extremities
11. Light bothers eyes (constantly need sunglasses)
12. Decrease volume when urinating
13. Heart pounds when trying to sleep
14. "Nervous" stomach
15. Reduced appetite
16. Cold sweats

17. Frequent fever
18. Numbness (where)
19. Habit of staring and not blinking
20. Frequent stomach aches
21. Morning joint stiffness
22. Leg cramps at night
23. Nervous stomach (butterflies)
24. Watery eyes or nose
25. Tendency to blink eyes often
26. Swollen eyes
27. Indigestion immediately after eating
28. Constantly feel hungry, often lightheaded
29. Frequent bouts of nausea and / or vomiting
30. Hoarseness or throat irritation
31. Irregular breathing or shortness of breath
32. Slow heart rate
33. Delayed gag reflex
34. Gags easily
35. Difficulty swallowing
36. Frequent need to clear throat
37. Constant "tickle" in throat
38. Alternate between loose stools and constipation
39. "Slow starter"
40. Perspire easily (list locations)
41. Sensitive to cold; poor circulation
42. Often catch colds
43. Asthmatic attacks or bouts of bronchitis
44. Nervous eater
45. Excessive appetite
46. Hungry between meals
47. Irritable before meals
48. Get "shaky" when hungry
49. Fatigue that is relieved by eating
50. Heart palpitations if meal is missed
51. Headaches in the afternoon
52. Digestive complaints if overeat sweets
53. Insomnia – difficulty falling asleep

54. Awaken after a few hours of sleep – difficulty falling back to sleep
55. Crave sugar or coffee in the afternoon
56. Bouts of depression or feeling melancholy
57. Excessive craving for sweets or snacks
58. Hands and feet "go to sleep" or become numb
59. Sigh frequently
60. Tendency to breathe heavy or gasp for air (trouble catching your breath)
61. Discomfort in high altitudes
62. Open windows in closed rooms
63. Subject to colds and fevers
64. Yawn frequently
65. Feel drowsy often
66. Swollen ankles that are worse at night
67. Muscle cramps especially during exercise- "charley horses"
68. Shortness of breath upon exertion
69. Lack of flexibility or complaints of tight muscles
70. Chronic dull chest pain often radiating into left arm (angina pain)
71. Bruise easily – often have inexplicable "black and blues"
72. History of anemia
73. Frequent nosebleeds
74. Ringing in ears (tinnitus)
75. Chronic chest tightness that is worse on exertion
76. Vertigo
77. Light-headed when standing
78. Jaw pain or "clicking"
79. Dry skin
80. Burning feet
81. Blurry vision
82. Itchy hands and feet
83. Excessive hair loss
84. Skin rashes
85. Bitter, metallic taste in mouth in the morning
86. Painful or difficult bowel movements
87. Worrier; feel insecure

88. Experience headaches over the eyes
89. Feeling of "queasiness"
90. Light colored stools
91. Black stools
92. Skin peels on the soles of the feet
93. Pain between the shoulder blades
94. Use of laxatives
95. Frequent diarrhea
96. History of gallstones or gallbladder attacks
97. Sneezing attacks
98. Frequent nightmares / disturbing dreams
99. Bad breath (halitosis)
100. Dairy products cause distress (lactose intolerance)
101. Sensitive to or an intolerance of hot weather
102. Burning or itchiness of the anus
103. Crave sweets
104. Lower body gas (flatulence) several hours after eating
105. Burning pain in stomach relieved by eating
106. Coated tongue
107. Indigestion up to 4 hours after eating
108. Mucous in stools
109. History of colitis or irritable bowel syndrome (IBS)
110. Gas or stomach bloating shortly after eating
111. Nervousness
112. Unable to gain weight
113. Unable to lose weight
114. Highly emotional
115. Blush easily
116. Night sweats
117. Sensation of trembling inside
118. Heart palpitations
119. Increased appetite with weight gain
120. Increased appetite without weight gain
121. Fast pulse even at rest
122. Eyelid and facial twitching
123. Irritable and restlessness
124. Quick temper

125. Unable to work under pressure
126. Inexplicable weight gain
127. Decrease in appetite
128. Fatigue easily
129. Constipation
130. Mental sluggishness
131. Hair becoming coarse and falling out
132. Headaches upon arising that fade as the day goes on
133. Frequent urination
134. Inexplicable loss or decrease of hearing
135. Visions problems
136. "Floaters" in the eye
137. Reduced initiative or drive to succeed
138. Memory diminishing
139. Low blood pressure
140. High blood pressure
141. Increased sex drive
142. Decreased sex drive
143. Severe "splitting" headaches
144. Dull headaches
145. Decrease tolerance for sugar
146. Excessive thirst
147. Abdominal bloating
148. Weight gain around hips or waist
149. Menstrual disorder or irregularities (female)
150. Lack of menstrual function (young females)
151. Infertility or miscarriages (female)
152. Hot flashes (females)
153. Hair growth on face or body (female)
154. Dizziness
155. Nails, weak or ridged
156. Hives
157. Arthritis or joint pains (show which joints on schematic)
158. Low back pain
159. Neck pain
160. Decreased perspiration (never sweat)
161. Crave salt

162. Brown spots or bronzing of skin
163. Allergies
164. Respiratory disorders (general)
165. Feeling of apprehension
166. Phobias
167. Easily forgetful
168. Difficulty focusing
169. Excessive muscular soreness
170. Sensitive to noises
171. Hearing disturbances (hear strange sounds)
172. Tendency to cry to no reason
173. Bouts of anxiety
174. Anorexia or bulimia
175. Leg nervousness at night (restless leg syndrome)
176. Infertility, prostate troubles or urination frequency/difficulties (men)
177. Migrating aches and pains
178. Feeling of incomplete bowel evacuation
179. Loss of strength (where)
180. Lack of energy

The AK specialist starts with this information and adds it to your prior medical records and diagnostic tests, along with information gleaned from speaking with you during your initial consultation. Once your personal profile is complete, the doctor will begin to implement AK examination procedures such as Gait and Postural Analysis—culminating with FMT to reveal the underlying cause of the condition or complaint.

RECOMMENDED READING

Blaich R. *Your Inner Pharmacy: Taking Back Our Wellness.* Hillsboro, OR: Beyond Words Publishing, Inc. 2006.

Callahan R, Trubo R. *Tapping the Healer Within: Using Thought-Field Therapy to Instantly Conquer Your Fears, Anxieties, and Emotional Distress.* New York, NY: McGraw-Hill, 2002.

Dean C. *The Magnesium Miracle.* New York, NY: Ballantine Books, 2017.

Diamond J. *Your Body Doesn't Lie.* New York, NY: Warner Books, Inc., 1979.

Force M. *Choosing Health: Dr. Force's Functional Selfcare Workbook.* Health Knowledge, 2003.

Fulford RC. *Touch of Life*, New York, NY: Simon & Schuster, 1996.

King S. *Live Without Pain: A New Theory on What's Wrong with You and How to Fix It.* UK: Naturality Press, 2008.

Maffetone P. *The Big Book of Endurance Training and Racing.* New York, NY: Skyhorse Publishing, 2010.

Maykel W. *The Tune Up: Hot Medicine for Everyone.* Wellness Medicine, 2017.

Mladenoff DV, Mladenoff E. *Stressed Out: Headed for Burnout.* Overland Park, KS: AIR Remedies, 2008.

Pert CB. *Molecules of Emotion.* New York, NY: Scribner, 1997.

Travell J. *Office Hours: Day and Night. The Autobiography of Janet Travell.* New York, NY: World Publishing Co., 1968.

NOTES

1. National Center for Health Statistics. Health, United States, 2017: With special feature on mortality. Hyattsville, MD. 2018
2. Medscape. "Medscape National Physician Burnout, Depression & Suicide Report 2019." https://www.medscape.com/slideshow/2019-lifestyle-burnout-depression-6011056 (accessed January 6, 2019).
3. "The World of Applied Kinesiology," https://icak.com (accessed December 25, 2018).
4. "International College of Applied Kinesiology® U.S.A," http://www.icakusa.com (accessed December 25, 2018).
5. Eugene Charles, "Applied Kinesiology: A Healthy Lifestyle Involves Movement, https://www.charlesseminars.com/doctorshome/ (accessed December 25, 2018).
6. Eugene Charles, "Applied Kinesiology Course Online—Dr. Charles Online," https://drcharlesonline.com (accessed December 25, 2018).
7. Jensen AM. Estimating the prevalence of use of kinesiology-style manual muscle testing: A survey of educators. *Advances in Integrative Medicine* 2015; 2(2): 96-102.
8. Pedersen BK. A muscular twist on the fate of fat. *The New England Journal of Medicine* 2012; 366(16): 1544-1545.
9. Boston P, Wu J, Jedrychowski MP, et a. A PGC1-α-dependent myokine that drives brown fat-like development of white fat and thermogenesis. *Nature* 2012; 481: 463-468.
10. Bishop B. Pain: its physiology and rationale for management. Part III. Consequences of current concepts of pain mechanisms

related to pain management. *Physical Therapy* 1980; 60(1): 24-37.

[11] Brel A. *Trail Guides to the Body: How to Locate Muscles, Bones, and More, 3rd Edition.* Boulder, CO: Books of Discovery, 2000.

[12] Rosner A, Leisman G, Gilchriest J, Charles E, Keschner M, Minond M. Reliability and validity of therapy localization as determined from multiple examiners and instrumentation. *Functional Neurology, Rehabilitation, and Ergonomics* 2015; 5(3): 365-386.

[13] Rosner AL, Charles E. Therapy localization in applied kinesiology: Validation by means of blinding in a cohort study. *Functional Neurology, Rehabilitation, and Ergonomics.* 2016; 6(2): 85-96.

[14] Center for Mindfulness in Medicine, Health Care, and Society. "Mindful Medicine: Relevance & Applications." www.instituteformindfulliving.com/instituteformindfulliving?Mindful Medicine.html (accessed January 9, 2019).

[15] Losina E, Thornhill TS, Rome BN, Wright J, Katz JN. The dramatic increase in total knee replacement utilization rates in the United States cannot be fully explained by growth in population size and the obesity epidemic. *Journal of Bone and Joint Surgery American* 2012; 94(3): 201-207.

[16] Orthopedics & Joint Care. Cape Regional Health System.com. https://www.caperegional.com/orthopaedicmedicine/joint-replacement-services (accessed December 26, 2016).

[17] American Academy of Orthopaedic Surgeons. 2.5 Million Americans Living with Artificial Hip, 4.7 Million with Artificial Knee. ScienceDaily.com https://www.sciencedaily.com/releases/2014/03/140314093737.htm (accessed December 26, 2018).

[18] Healthcare Cost and Utilization Project (HCUP). Agency for Healthcare Research and Quality, Rockville, MD. http://hcupnet.ahrq.gov (accessed December 27, 2018).

[19] Stanford Center for Continuing Medical Education: 25 Bedside Medicine Symposium, September 29-30, 2017, Stanford, CA. https://med.stanfordedu/cme/course/2017/stan25html (accessed January 6, 2019).

[20] Hoy D, March L, Brooks P, Flyth F, Woolf A, et al. The global burden of low back pain: estimates from the Global Burden of Disease 2010 study. *Annals of the Rheumatic Diseases* 2014; 73: 968-974.

[21] Langlois JA, Rutland-Brown W, Wald MM. The epidemiology and impact of traumatic brain injury: a brief overview. *Journal of Head Trauma and Rehabilitation* 2006; 21(5): 375-378.

[22] National Safety Council. "Concussion Care Should Top Every Youth Sports Playbook. https://www.nsc.org/home-safety.concussions (accessed December 30, 2018).

[23] PR in Motion News. "CDC: Concussion Rates Among High Schoolers May be Undercounted." www.apta.org/PTinMotiion/News/2018/06/25/CDC/ConcussionsHighSchool/ (accessed December 30, 2018).

[24] Sports Concussion Statistics. Headcase.com. www.headcasecompany.com/concussion_info/stats._on_concussion (accessed December 30, 2018).

[25] UPMC Health Beat. "Concussion and Loss of Consciousness" https://share.upmc.com/2015/04/concussion-and-loss-of-consciousness/ (accessed December 30, 2018).

[26] Brain Injury Association of America. "Brain Trauma Indicator Blood Test Approved by FDA. https://www.biausa.org/public-affairs/public-awareness/news/brain-trauma-indicator-test-approved-by-fda (accessed December 30, 2018).

[27] Brooks M. "FDA Clears Novel Eye Tracking Device to Detect Concussion." Medscape January 10, 2019. https://www.medscape.com/viewarticle/907366?nlid=127114_3901&src=wnl_newsalrt_190108_MSCPEDIT&uac=129669BT&impID=1855110&faf=1 (accessed January 10, 2019).

[28] Naples Neurosurgery. "Whiplash Injury." https://neurosurgeon.com/conditions/whiplash/ (accessed January 6, 2019).

[29] Healthline. "GERD: Facts, Statistics, and You." https://www.healthline.com/health/cerd/facts-statistics-infographc#1 (accessed January 6, 2019).

[30] National Digestive Diseases Information Clearinghouse. Constipation. NIH Publication No. 13-2754, September 2013.

sfsurgery.com/wp-content/uploads/2014/06/Constipation.pdf (accessed December 30, 2014).

[31] Sommers T, Corban C, Sengupta N, Jones M, Cheng V, Bollom A, Nurko S, Kelley J, Lembo A. Emergency department burden of constipation in the United States from 2006 to 2011. *American Journal of Gastroenterology* 2015; 110(4): 572-579.

[32] Schmier JK, Miller PE, Levine JA, Perez VY, Maki KC, Rains TM, Devareddy L, Sanders LM, Alexander DD. Cost savings of reduced constipation rates attributed to increased dietary fiber intakes: A decision-analytic model. *BMC Public Health* 2014; 14(1): 374.

33 American Heart Association. "Heart, How It Works." www.heart.org/HEARTORG/Affiliate/Heart-How-It-Works_UCM_428843.Artic;le.jsp#XCp8mM17mUk (accessed 12/31/2018).

[34] World Health Organization. "Global Report on Diabetes." https://www.who.int/diabetes/en/ (accessed December 31, 2018).

[35] International Diabetes Federation. "About Diabetes." www.https://www.idf.org/aboutdiabetes/what-is-diabetes/facts-figures.html (accessed December 31, 2018).

[36] Centers for Disease Control and Prevention. "CDC Newsroom: New CDC Report: More than 100 Million Americans Have Diabetes or Prediabetes." https://www.cdc.gov/media/releases/2017/p07-18-diabetes-report.html (accessed December 31, 2018).

[37] Thyroid Foundation of Canada. "About thyroid disease." http://thyroid.ca/thyroid-disease (accessed March 2017).

[38] American Thyroid Association. "General Information/Press Room." https://www.thyroid.org/media-main/press-room/ (accessed December 31, 2018).

[39] Schiefer M, Teixeira PFS, Fontenelle C, Carminatti T, Santos DA, Righi LD, Conceicao EL. Prevalence of hypothyroidism in patients with frozen shoulder. *Journal of Shoulder and Elbow Surgery* 2017; 26(1): 49-55.

[40] United States Environmental Protection Agency. The EPA Blog. "How Many Breaths Do You Take Each Day?" https://

blog.epa.gov/2014/04/28/how-many-breathes-do-you-take-each-day/ (accessed January 1, 2019).

[41] Discovery Health. "How Much Oxygen Does a Person Consume in a Day?" https:/www.sharecar.com/health/air-quality/oxygen-person-consume-a-day (accessed January 1, 2019).

[42] Ochs M, Nyengaard JR, Jung A, Knudsen L, Voigt M, Wahlers T, Richter J, Gundersen HJG. The number of alveoli in the human lung. *America Journal of Respiratory and Critical Care Medicine* 2004; 169(1): 120-124.

[43] Asher I, Pearce N. Global burden of asthma among children. *International Journal of Tuberculosis and Lung Diseases* 2014; 18(11): 1269-1278.

[44] Centers for Disease Control and Prevention. "Asthma in the United States, June 2014." http://www.cdc.gov/asthma/asthma_prevalance_in_us.pptx. (accessed January 1, 2019).

[45] American Lung Association. Lung Health & Diseases. "Asthma Risk Factors" https://www.lung.org/lung-health-and-diseases/lung-disease-lookup/asthma/asthma-symptoms-causes-risk-factors/asthma-risk-factors.html. (accessed January 1, 2019).

[46] World Health Organization. "Headache Disorders" https://www/who.int/news-room/fact-sheets/detail/headache-disorders (accessed January 1, 2019).

[47] Migraine Research Foundation. "Migraine Facts." http://migraineresearchfoundation.org/about-migraine/migraine-facts/ (accessed February 21, 2018).

[48] Victor TW, Hu X, Campbell JC, et al. Migraine prevalence by age and sex in the United States: a life-span study. *Cephalalgia* 2010; 30: 1065-1072.

[49] American Migraine Foundation. "Tension-Type Headaches: The Basics" https://americanmigrainefoundation.org/resource-library/tension-type-headache/ (accessed January 1, 2019).

[50] Brooks M. "FDA OKs Vagus Nerve Stimulator to Prevent Cluster Headaches." Medscape Business Medicine. https://www.medscape.com/viewarticle/905929?src=WNL_infoc_190111/MSCPEDIT_TEMP2&uac=1296698T&impID=1857026&faf=1 (accessed January 12, 2019).

[51] Encyclopedia Britannica. "Physiology" https://www.britannica.com/science/information-theory/Physiology (accessed January 2, 2019).

[52] Centers for Disease Control and Prevention. "Attention-Deficit/Hyperactivity Disorder (ADHD)" https://www.cdc.gov/ncbddd/adhd/features/key-findings-adhd72013.html (accessed January 2, 2019).

[53] Riccio CA, Wolfe M, Davis B, Romaine C, George C, Lee D. Attention deficit hyperactivity disorder: manifestation in adulthood. *Archives of Clinical Neuropsychology* 2005; 20(2): 249-269.

[54] Allahdadi KJ, Tostes RCA, Webb RC. Female sexual dysfunction: Therapeutic options and experimental challenges. *Cardiovascular & Hematological Agents in Medicinal Chemistry* 2009; 7(4): 260-269.

[55] Erectile dysfunction in older men. *Consultant* 2010; 18(7): https://www.consultant360.com/articleserectile-dysfunction-older-men (accessed January 2, 2019).

[56] Eunice Kennedy Shriver National Institute of Child Health and Human Development. "How Common Is Infertility? https://www.nichd.nih.gov/health/topics/infertility/conditionsinfo/common (accessed January 2, 2019).

[57] Lakin M, Wood H. Erectile dysfunction. Cleveland Clinic Center for Continuing Education. June 2018. www.clevelandclinicmeded.com/medicalpubs/diseasemanagement/endocrinology/erectile-dysfunction (accessed January 3, 2019).

[58] ABC News. "1 in 4 Men Over 30 Has Low Testosterone." https://abcnews.go.com/Health/Healthday/story?id=45086698page=1 (accessed January 6, 2019).

[59] Medscape. "Varicocele" https://emedicine.medscape.com/article/438591-overview (accessed January 3, 2019).

[60] Centers for Disease Control and Prevention. "Gateway to Health Communication & Social Marketing Practice. Allergies." www.cdc.gov/healthcommunication/toolstemplates/entertamimented/tips/Allergies.html (accessed January 3, 2019).

[61] Pawankar R, Canonica WG, Holgate ST, Lockey RF. *White Book on Allergy 2011-2012 Executive Summary.*

[62] Schoenwetter WF, Dupclay L Jr, Appajosyula S, et al. Economic impact and quality-of-life burden of allergic rhinitis. *Current Medical Research and Opinion* 2004; 20(3): 305-317.

RESOURCES

Conable K, Corneal J, Hambrick T, Marquina N, Zhang J. Investigation of methods and styles of manual muscle testing by AK practitioners. *Journal of Chiropractic Medicine* 2010; 1(4): 1-10.

Cuthbert SC, Goodheart GJ Jr. On the reliability and validity of manual muscle testing: a literature review. *Chiropractic & Osteopathy* 2007; 15(1): 4.

Cuthbert S, Lindley-Jones S. A history of professional applied kinesiology around the world. *International Journal of Functional Manual Muscle Testing*. December 2018.

Cuthbert SC, Rosner A, McDowall D. Association of manual muscle tests and mechanical neck pain: results from a prospective pilot study. *Journal of Bodywork and Movement Therapies*; 2011: 15: 192-200.

Goodheart GJ. Muscle strength testing as a diagnostic screen for supplemental nutrition therapy: letter to the Editor. *Journal of Manipulative and Physiological Therapeutics* 1983; 6(2): 87.

Goodheart GJ. Applied kinesiology: what does the term mean? Letter to the Editor. *Journal of the American Dietary Association* 1988; 89(4): 477.

Hall S, Lewith G, Brien S, Little P. A review of the literature in applied and specialized kinesiology. *Forschende Komplementarmedizin 2008; 15(1): 40-46.*

Janda V. On the concept of postural muscles and posture in man. *Australian Journal of Physiotherapy* 1983; 29: 83-84.

Janda V, Frank C, Liebenson C. Evaluation of muscle imbalance. *In* Liebenson C (Ed.) *Rehabilitation of the Spine, 2nd Edition.* Baltimore, MD: Williams & Wilkins, 2006; pp. 203-225.

Kendall FP, McCreary EK, Provance PG, Rodgers MM, Romani WA. *Muscles, Testing and Function with Posture and Pain.* Baltimore, MD: Williams & Wilkins, 2005.

Leaf D. Severe equilibrium problems non-responsive to pharmacological care treated with Chiropractic and applied kinesiology: a case history. *International Journal of Kinesiological Medicine* 2002; 13: 27.

Leisman G, Zenhausem R, Ferentz A, Tefera T, Zemcov A. Electromyographic effects of fatigue and task repetition on the validity of estimates of strong and weak muscles in applied kinesiological muscle-testing procedures. *Perceptual and Motor Skills* 1995; 80: 963-977.

Levit K. *Manipulative Therapy in Rehabilitation of the Locomotor System, 3rd Edition.* London: Butterworths, 1999.

Melczak JR, Wall PD. *The Puzzle of Pain*, 1973: New York, NY: Basic Books

Mladenoff DV, Mladenoff E. *Stressed Out: Headed for Burnout.* Overland Park, KS: AIR Remedies, 2008.

Moncayo R, Moncayo H. Evaluation of applied kinesiology meridian techniques by means of surface electromyography (EMG): demonstration of the regulatory influence of antique acupuncture points. *Chinese Medicine* 2004; 10(4): 643-650.

Pollard HP, Bablis P, Bonello R. The ileocecal valve point and muscle testing: a possible mechanism of action. *Chiropractic Journal of Australia* 2006; 36(4): 122-126.

Rosner AL, Cuthbert SC. Applied kinesiology: Distinctions in its definition and interpretation. *Journal of Bodywork and Movement Therapies* 2012; 16(1): 42-49.

Schmitt WH, Cuthbert SC. Common errors and clinical guidelines for manual muscle testing. The “arm test” and other inaccurate procedures. *Chiropractic & Osteopathy* 2008; 16: 16.

Schmitt WH, Leisman G. Correlation of applied kinesiology muscle testing findings with serum immunoglobulin levels for food allergies. *International Journal of Neuroscience* 1998; 96(3-4): 237-244.

Schmitt WH JR., Yanuck SF. Expanding the neurological examination using functional neurological assessment. Part II: Neurological basis of Applied Kinesiology. *International Journal of Neuroscience* 1998; 97(1-2).

Walther DS. Applied Kinesiology Synopsis, 2nd Edition. Shawnee Mission, KS: International College of Applied Kinesiology, 2000.

WHERE TO LEARN APPLIED KINESIOLOGY

Health care practitioners who are interested in implementing Applied Kinesiology into their practices can take courses from:

1. The International College of Applied Kinesiology (ICAK) for live classes at www.icak.com or www.icakusa.com (913) 384-5336
2. Charles Seminars for DVD and online classes at: www.charlesseminars.com or www.drcharlesonline.com (800) 351-5450

You are eligible for a tuition discount from the Online Course by typing JTH when you register

CPSIA information can be obtained
at www.ICGtesting.com
Printed in the USA
BVHW031926310319
544176BV00004B/9/P